Diabetic Air Fryer Cookbook 2024

1700 Days of Easy, Healthy Low-Fat Recipes for Type 1 & 2 Diabetes with a 28-Day Meal Plan and 4-Week Shopping List

Contents

Introduction... 4

Understanding Diabetes and Diet........................... 5

How to Use This Cookbook 8

1 Mastering Your Air Fryer 9

2 Diabetes Insights 13

3 Breakfast Recipes 18

4 Morning Snack Recipes.. 29

5 Lunch Recipes... 40

6 Afternoon Snack Recipes.................................... 53

7 Dinner Recipes 64

8 Dessert Recipes... 79

9 28-Day Meal Plan 89

10 Shopping List for 4-Week Meal Plan 94

Conclusion 100

Air Fryer Cooking Chart 102

Kitchen Measurements Conversion Chart 103

Bonus Book...104

Recipes Index.. 105

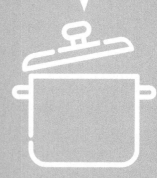

Introduction

Welcome to Your Healthier Kitchen

Welcome to the "Diabetic Air Fryer Cookbook 2024: 1700 Days of Easy, Healthy Low-Fat Recipes for Type 1 & 2 Diabetes with a 28-Day Meal Plan." This cookbook is designed to be your comprehensive guide to achieving and maintaining balanced wellness through delicious, diabetes-friendly meals prepared with the convenience and health benefits of an air fryer.

Living with diabetes can often feel like a constant balancing act. Managing your blood sugar levels, making mindful food choices, and maintaining a healthy lifestyle can be overwhelming. This book aims to simplify that process by providing you with a wealth of recipes and meal plans that are not only healthy but also incredibly tasty and easy to prepare.

The air fryer is a game-changer in the kitchen, allowing you to enjoy all your favorite fried foods with significantly less oil. This means you can indulge in crispy, mouthwatering dishes without the guilt or the negative health impacts associated with traditional frying methods. The recipes in this cookbook are specifically designed to be low-fat, low-carb, and low-sugar, making them ideal for managing diabetes without sacrificing flavor or variety.

Understanding Diabetes and Diet

What is Diabetes?

Diabetes is a chronic health condition that affects how your body turns food into energy. It involves issues with insulin, a hormone made by the pancreas that helps glucose from food get into your cells to be used for energy. When insulin is not produced effectively or the body cannot use it properly, glucose stays in your bloodstream, leading to high blood sugar levels. Over time, this can cause serious health problems.

There are two main types of diabetes:

Type 1 Diabetes: This is an autoimmune condition where the body's immune system attacks the insulin-producing cells in the pancreas. People with Type 1 diabetes need to take insulin every day to manage their blood sugar levels. It is usually diagnosed in children, teens, and young adults but can develop at any age.

Type 2 Diabetes: This is the most common type of diabetes. It occurs when the body becomes resistant to insulin or when the pancreas doesn't produce enough insulin. It is often associated with older age, obesity, family history, and physical inactivity. Type 2 diabetes can often be managed with lifestyle changes, but medications or insulin therapy may also be needed.

The Importance of Diet in Diabetes Management

Diet plays a crucial role in managing diabetes. The food you eat can directly impact your blood sugar levels, so making informed dietary choices is essential. Here's why diet is so important:

Blood Sugar Control: Different foods have varying effects on blood glucose levels. Carbohydrates, for example, have the most significant impact because they are broken down into glucose. Understanding how different foods affect your blood sugar can help you manage it more effectively.

Weight Management: Maintaining a healthy weight is vital for managing Type 2 diabetes. Excess weight, particularly around the abdomen, can increase insulin resistance. A balanced diet can help you achieve and maintain a healthy weight.

Preventing Complications: Consistently high blood sugar levels can lead to complications such as heart disease, kidney damage, and nerve damage. A healthy diet helps keep blood sugar levels within a target range, reducing the risk of these complications.

Key Dietary Principles for Managing Diabetes

Carbohydrate Management
Carbohydrates are a primary source of energy, but they have the most significant impact on blood sugar levels. Understanding carbohydrate counting and choosing the right types of carbohydrates can help you manage your diabetes more effectively.

Complex Carbohydrates: Foods such as whole grains, legumes, and vegetables contain complex carbohydrates. They are digested more slowly, causing a slower and more gradual rise in blood sugar levels.

Simple Carbohydrates: Foods such as sugary drinks, candies, and white bread contain simple carbohydrates. They are quickly digested and can cause rapid spikes in blood sugar levels.

Glycemic Index (GI)

The glycemic index is a measure of how quickly a food causes your blood sugar levels to rise. Foods with a high GI are rapidly digested and cause a quick spike in blood sugar, while foods with a low GI are digested more slowly and cause a gradual rise in blood sugar.

Low GI Foods: Whole grains, legumes, most fruits, and non-starchy vegetables.

High GI Foods: White bread, white rice, potatoes, and sugary snacks.

Balanced Diet

A balanced diet includes a variety of foods from all food groups in the right proportions. This helps ensure you get all the necessary nutrients without consuming too many calories or unhealthy fats.

Fruits and Vegetables: Aim to fill half your plate with fruits and vegetables. They are low in calories and high in fiber, vitamins, and minerals.

Protein: Include lean proteins such as fish, chicken, beans, and nuts. Protein helps build and repair tissues and does not cause a spike in blood sugar levels.

Fats: Choose healthy fats such as those found in avocados, nuts, seeds, and olive oil. Avoid trans fats and limit saturated fats.

Portion Control

Eating the right portions is crucial for managing diabetes. Overeating, even healthy foods, can lead to weight gain and increased blood sugar levels. Using smaller plates, measuring your food, and being mindful of your eating habits can help control portions.

Regular Meal Times

Eating at regular times each day helps control blood sugar levels. Skipping meals or having irregular meal times can cause blood sugar levels to fluctuate significantly. Aim for three balanced meals a day with healthy snacks in between if needed.

Specific Dietary Recommendations for Diabetics

Fiber-Rich Foods

Fiber slows down the absorption of sugar and helps improve blood sugar levels. It also aids in digestion and can help you feel full, which is beneficial for weight management. Include plenty of vegetables, fruits, legumes, and whole grains in your diet.

Stay Hydrated

Drinking plenty of water is essential for everyone, but especially for people with diabetes. It helps regulate blood sugar levels and can prevent dehydration. Aim to drink at least 8 glasses of water a day.

Limit Alcohol

If you choose to drink alcohol, do so in moderation. Alcohol can cause blood sugar levels to drop or spike, depending on how much you drink and if you consume it with food. Always check your blood sugar levels before and after drinking.

Reduce Sodium Intake

High sodium intake can lead to high blood pressure, which is a risk factor for cardiovascular disease, a common complication of diabetes. Limit processed foods and use herbs and spices to flavor your food instead of salt.

Sample Daily Meal Plan

Here's a sample meal plan to give you an idea of how to structure your meals for a day:

Breakfast: Greek yogurt with berries and a sprinkle of chia seeds, a slice of whole-grain toast with avocado.

Morning Snack: A small apple with a handful of almonds.

Lunch: Grilled chicken salad with mixed greens, cherry tomatoes, cucumber, and a vinaigrette dressing.

Afternoon Snack: Carrot sticks with hummus.

Dinner: Baked salmon with a side of quinoa and steamed broccoli.

Dessert: A small serving of mixed berries.

How to Use This Cookbook

This cookbook is structured to make your culinary journey as smooth and enjoyable as possible. Here's how you can make the most of it:

Start with the Basics: If you are new to using an air fryer, begin with Chapter 1, where you'll find all the essential tips and tricks to get you started. Learn how to use, maintain, and master your air fryer to create perfect meals every time.

Understand Your Health Needs: Chapter 2 provides valuable insights into diabetes and nutrition. Understanding the relationship between food and your blood sugar levels will empower you to make informed choices.

Explore the Recipes: Dive into the extensive collection of recipes organized by meal type. Whether you're looking for a quick breakfast, a hearty lunch, a satisfying dinner, or a guilt-free dessert, you'll find plenty of options to suit your taste and dietary needs.

Follow the Meal Plan: a comprehensive 28-day meal plan is included in the book to guide you through a month of healthy eating. This plan is designed to simplify your daily decision-making and ensure you get a balanced variety of nutrients.

Take Advantage of Bonus Content: Don't miss the bonus sections that include additional guides and tips to further support your journey. From mastering the air fryer to understanding diabetes in depth and making smart dining-out choices, these extras are here to enhance your experience.

Conclusion

Managing diabetes through diet doesn't mean you have to sacrifice flavor or enjoyment. By understanding the impact of different foods on your blood sugar levels and making informed dietary choices, you can enjoy a variety of delicious meals while keeping your diabetes under control. The "Diabetic Air Fryer Cookbook 2024" is here to guide you on this journey, providing you with easy, healthy, and tasty recipes that support your health and well-being. Embrace the power of nutritious ingredients, simplify your meal preparation, and savor the flavors of a healthy lifestyle.

Getting Started with Your Air Fryer

The air fryer has revolutionized the way we cook, offering a healthier alternative to traditional frying methods. By circulating hot air around food, it creates a crispy, fried texture with significantly less oil. This makes it an ideal cooking method for those managing diabetes, as it helps reduce fat intake without sacrificing flavor or texture. In this chapter, we'll cover everything you need to know to get started with your air fryer, from setup and maintenance to mastering the cooking techniques that will make your meals both delicious and healthy.

What is an Air Fryer?

An air fryer is a countertop kitchen appliance that cooks by circulating hot air around food. It uses a convection mechanism to cook the food quickly and evenly, producing a crispy layer similar to traditional frying but with much less oil. This not only makes the food healthier but also cuts down on the cooking time and the mess associated with deep frying.

Types of Air Fryers

1. **Basket/Bucket Style Air Fryers:** These are the most common types, featuring a pull-out basket where food is placed. They are great for preparing fried foods like French fries, chicken wings, and fish sticks.

2. **Oven-Style Air Fryers:** These air fryers look similar to a countertop convection oven and often have multiple racks, allowing you to cook larger quantities of food or multiple dishes at once. They are perfect for baking, roasting, and dehydrating.

3. **Paddle-Type Air Fryers:** These come with a paddle that stirs the food automatically, ensuring even cooking without manual shaking or turning. They are ideal for dishes that need constant movement, such as stir-fries and risottos.

4. **Toaster Oven Air Fryers:** Combining the functions of a toaster oven and an air fryer, these appliances are highly versatile and can perform a variety of cooking tasks, from toasting and baking to air frying and broiling.

Benefits of Using an Air Fryer

- **Healthier Cooking:** Air fryers require little to no oil, reducing the fat content of traditionally fried foods, which is beneficial for managing diabetes and overall health.
- **Convenience:** They cook food faster than conventional ovens and are easy to clean.
- **Versatility:** Air fryers can cook a wide variety of foods, from vegetables and meats to desserts and snacks.
- **Consistent Results:** With proper use, air fryers can deliver consistent, crispy, and evenly cooked results.
- **Weight Management:** Lower fat content in meals can help with weight management, an essential aspect of managing Type 2 diabetes.
- **Blood Sugar Control:** Using an air fryer to cook low-carb, low-sugar meals helps maintain stable blood sugar levels.

Benefits of Air Frying for Diabetes Management and Health

1. **Lower Fat Intake:** Traditional frying methods often involve large amounts of oil, which can add unnecessary fat and calories to your diet. Air frying significantly

reduces the need for oil, helping to lower your overall fat intake. This is crucial for diabetes management, as a diet high in unhealthy fats can lead to insulin resistance and exacerbate Type 2 diabetes.

2. **Improved Heart Health:** Reduced fat intake also contributes to better heart health. High cholesterol levels are common in people with diabetes, and lowering your fat intake can help manage cholesterol levels, reducing the risk of cardiovascular diseases.

3. **Better Weight Management:** Air frying aids in maintaining a healthy weight by reducing calorie intake from fats. Maintaining a healthy weight is essential for managing diabetes and preventing complications.

4. **Consistent Blood Sugar Levels:** Air fryers can help prepare meals that are lower in carbohydrates and sugars, which are essential for keeping blood sugar levels stable. Cooking methods that involve less oil and fat also help in maintaining a lower glycemic index, making it easier to control blood sugar spikes.

5. **Enhanced Nutritional Value:** Air frying preserves more nutrients compared to other cooking methods like deep frying or boiling, which can destroy vitamins and minerals. This ensures that your meals are not only delicious but also packed with essential nutrients that support overall health and diabetes management.

Setting Up Your Air Fryer

1. **Unboxing and Inspection**
- Remove all packaging materials and stickers from your air fryer.
- Inspect the unit for any damage or missing parts.
- Read the user manual thoroughly to familiarize yourself with the appliance's features and functions.

2. **Placement**
- Place the air fryer on a flat, stable, and heat-resistant surface.
- Ensure there is sufficient space around the air fryer for ventilation. Avoid placing it near walls or other appliances.

3. **Initial Cleaning**
- Wash the basket, tray, and any removable parts with warm, soapy water.
- Wipe the interior and exterior of the air fryer with a damp cloth.
- Allow all parts to dry completely before reassembling.

4. **Initial Test Run**
- Plug in the air fryer and turn it on.
- Run it empty at a high temperature (around 400°F or 200°C) for 10-15 minutes. This helps to burn off any residual oils or manufacturing residues.

Understanding the Controls

Air fryers come with various control options, including digital and manual settings. Here's a general overview of the controls you might find:

- **Temperature Control:** Allows you to set the cooking temperature, typically ranging from 180°F to 400°F (80°C to 200°C).
- **Timer:** Sets the cooking time, usually up to 60 minutes.
- **Preset Programs:** Many air fryers have preset cooking programs for common foods like fries, chicken, fish, and baked goods.
- **Start/Stop Button:** Begins or stops the cooking process.
- **Shake Reminder:** Some models include a reminder to shake or turn the food halfway through the cooking process for even cooking.

Tips and Tricks for Air Frying Success

1. Preheat Your Air Fryer
- Preheating ensures that the air fryer reaches the desired temperature before you add your food, resulting in more even cooking. Preheat for 3-5 minutes at the temperature specified in your recipe.

2. Do Not Overcrowd the Basket
- Overcrowding can prevent proper air circulation, leading to uneven cooking. Cook food in batches if necessary to ensure each piece gets crispy and evenly cooked.

3. Use Oil Sparingly
- While air fryers require less oil than traditional frying, a light coating of oil can enhance crispiness. Use a spray bottle to lightly mist food with oil or toss it in a small amount of oil before cooking.

4. Shake or Turn Food
- For even cooking, shake the basket or turn the food halfway through the cooking process. This is especially important for smaller items like fries or chicken nuggets.

5. Experiment with Seasoning
- Enhance the flavor of your dishes by experimenting with different herbs and spices. Add seasoning before and after cooking to achieve the best flavor.

6. Use Parchment Paper or Foil
- For easier cleanup, line the basket with parchment paper or aluminum foil. Make sure to leave space for air to circulate.

7. Check Food Early
- Air fryers cook quickly, so check your food a few minutes before the recommended cooking time to avoid overcooking.

Cleaning and Maintenance

1. After Each Use
- Allow the air fryer to cool completely before cleaning.
- Remove and wash the basket, tray, and any other removable parts with warm, soapy water.
- Wipe down the interior and exterior of the air fryer with a damp cloth. Do not use abrasive sponges or harsh chemicals.

2. Weekly Maintenance
- Inspect the heating element for any buildup or residue. Wipe it clean if necessary.
- Check the air intake and exhaust vents for any blockages and clean them to ensure proper airflow.

3. Deep Cleaning
- For a thorough cleaning, soak the basket and tray in warm, soapy water for 10-15 minutes before scrubbing.
- Use a soft brush to clean any hard-to-reach areas.
- If your air fryer has a non-stick coating, be gentle to avoid damaging it.

Troubleshooting Common Issues

1. Uneven Cooking
- Ensure the basket is not overcrowded.
- Shake or turn the food halfway through cooking.

2. Food Not Crispy
- Increase the temperature slightly.
- Lightly coat the food with oil.

3. Smoke Emission
- Excess oil or food residue can cause smoke. Clean the basket and tray thoroughly.
- Avoid cooking fatty foods at very high temperatures.

4. Air Fryer Not Heating
- Check that the appliance is plugged in securely.
- Ensure the basket is properly inserted.
- Consult the user manual for specific troubleshooting steps.

Conclusion

Mastering your air fryer opens up a world of healthy and delicious cooking possibilities. By understanding the basics of setup, maintenance, and cooking techniques, you can make the most of this versatile appliance. Whether you're preparing a quick snack or a full meal, the air fryer can help you achieve crispy, flavorful results with minimal effort and oil. With the added benefits of better diabetes management, improved heart health, and enhanced nutritional value, the air fryer is a valuable tool in your journey to healthier eating. With the tips and tricks provided in this chapter, you'll be well on your way to becoming an air frying expert, ready to tackle the delicious and diabetes-friendly recipes in this cookbook.

Chapter 2: Diabetes Insights

Managing diabetes effectively requires a comprehensive understanding of the condition and how various factors, including diet, exercise, and medication, impact blood sugar levels. This chapter delves into the intricacies of diabetes, offering insights into its types, the importance of glycemic index, the role of nutrition, and strategies for maintaining balanced blood sugar levels. Additionally, it provides guidance on combining a diabetic diet with air frying to optimize health and flavor.

Understanding Diabetes

Diabetes is a chronic condition that affects how your body processes glucose, a vital source of energy derived from food. There are three primary types of diabetes: Type 1, Type 2, and gestational diabetes. Each type has unique characteristics and management needs.

1. **Type 1 Diabetes**
- **Definition:** An autoimmune condition where the immune system attacks and destroys insulin-producing beta cells in the pancreas.
- **Diagnosis:** Often diagnosed in childhood or adolescence but can occur at any age.
- **Management:** Requires daily insulin injections or an insulin pump, along with regular blood sugar monitoring and a balanced diet.

2. **Type 2 Diabetes**
- **Definition:** A condition characterized by insulin resistance and relative insulin deficiency. The body cannot use insulin effectively, leading to elevated blood sugar levels.
- **Diagnosis:** Typically diagnosed in adults over 45, but increasing numbers of children, adolescents, and younger adults are developing it.

- **Management:** Managed through lifestyle changes such as diet and exercise, oral medications, and sometimes insulin.

3. **Gestational Diabetes**
- **Definition:** A form of diabetes that develops during pregnancy and usually resolves after childbirth.
- **Diagnosis:** Occurs in pregnant women who have never had diabetes before.
- **Management:** Managed through diet, exercise, and sometimes insulin. Monitoring is crucial to prevent complications for both mother and baby.

The Importance of Glycemic Index

The glycemic index (GI) is a ranking system for carbohydrates based on their effect on blood glucose levels. Foods with a high GI are rapidly digested and absorbed, causing a quick rise in blood sugar levels. Foods with a low GI are digested more slowly, resulting in a gradual rise in blood sugar.

1. **Low GI Foods**
- **Examples:** Whole grains, legumes, most fruits, and non-starchy vegetables.
- **Benefits:** Help maintain steady blood sugar levels and reduce insulin spikes. They also promote satiety, which can aid in weight management.

2. **High GI Foods**
- **Examples:** White bread, white rice, potatoes, and sugary snacks.
- **Drawbacks:** Cause rapid spikes in blood sugar, which can lead to insulin resistance over time. They may also contribute to increased hunger and overeating.

3. **Using GI for Meal Planning**
- **Balancing Meals:** Combine low GI foods with moderate or high GI foods to balance the overall GI of a meal.
- **Portion Control:** Be mindful of portion sizes, even with low GI foods, to avoid excessive calorie intake.

The Role of Nutrition in Diabetes Management

A balanced diet is fundamental to managing diabetes. Proper nutrition helps regulate blood sugar levels, manage weight, and reduce the risk of complications such as heart disease and neuropathy.

1. **Carbohydrates**
- **Types:** Simple carbohydrates (sugars) and complex carbohydrates (starches and fiber).
- **Impact:** Carbohydrates have the most significant impact on blood sugar levels. Understanding carbohydrate counting and choosing the right types can help manage diabetes effectively.

2. **Proteins**
- **Sources:** Lean meats, poultry, fish, eggs, dairy, legumes, and plant-based proteins.
- **Role:** Protein helps build and repair tissues, and it has a minimal impact on blood sugar levels. Including protein in meals can promote satiety and stabilize blood sugar.

3. **Fats**
- **Types:** Saturated fats, trans fats, monounsaturated fats, and polyunsaturated fats.
- **Impact:** Healthy fats (monounsaturated and polyunsaturated) are beneficial for heart health, which is crucial for people with diabetes. Limit intake of saturated and trans fats to reduce the risk of cardiovascular diseases.

4. **Fiber**
- **Sources:** Fruits, vegetables, whole grains, legumes, nuts, and seeds.
- **Benefits:** Fiber slows down the absorption of sugar, helping to regulate blood sugar levels. It also aids in digestion and can help with weight management.

5. **Vitamins and Minerals**
- **Importance:** Essential for overall health and well-being. People with diabetes should ensure they get adequate amounts of vitamins and minerals through a varied diet or supplements if needed.

Combining a Diabetic Diet with Air Frying

Air frying can be an excellent method to prepare diabetes-friendly meals. It reduces the amount of oil needed for cooking, helping to lower fat and calorie intake, which is crucial for managing diabetes. Here's how to integrate air frying into a diabetic diet:

1. **Choosing the Right Foods**
- Opt for lean proteins like chicken, fish, and tofu, which can be air-fried to perfection with minimal oil.
- Select non-starchy vegetables such as broccoli, cauliflower, bell peppers, and zucchini for air frying. These vegetables are low in carbs and high in fiber.
- Use whole grains like quinoa and brown rice as side dishes to complement your air-fried main courses.

2. **Using Healthy Oils**
- Use heart-healthy oils such as olive oil, avocado oil, or canola oil in small amounts. A light spray or brushing is sufficient for air frying.
- Avoid oils high in saturated and trans fats, which can negatively impact heart health.

3. **Seasoning for Flavor**
- Enhance the flavor of your dishes with herbs

and spices instead of relying on salt and sugar. Ingredients like garlic, rosemary, paprika, and cumin can add depth to your meals without affecting blood sugar levels.

4. Portion Control
- Air frying allows you to prepare just the right amount of food, helping to avoid overeating. Pay attention to serving sizes to ensure balanced meals.

5. Incorporating Low GI Foods
- Combine air-fried dishes with low GI foods to keep your meals balanced. For instance, pair air-fried chicken with a salad of leafy greens and a side of quinoa.

6. Experimenting with Recipes
- Explore a variety of recipes to keep your meals interesting and enjoyable. Try air-fried salmon with a lemon-dill sauce or air-fried eggplant with a light tomato basil topping.

Strategies for Maintaining Balanced Blood Sugar Levels

1. Regular Monitoring
- **Frequency:** Check blood sugar levels regularly as advised by your healthcare provider.
- **Tools:** Use a blood glucose meter or continuous glucose monitor (CGM) for accurate readings.
- **Benefits:** Helps track how food, exercise, and medications affect blood sugar levels, allowing for timely adjustments.

2. Meal Timing and Frequency
- **Consistency:** Eat meals and snacks at regular intervals to avoid large fluctuations in blood sugar levels.
- **Balance:** Include a mix of carbohydrates, proteins, and fats in each meal to promote stable blood sugar levels.

3. Physical Activity
- **Benefits:** Exercise improves insulin sensitivity, helps manage weight, and reduces blood sugar levels.
- **Types:** Aim for a combination of aerobic exercises (such as walking, cycling, or swimming) and strength training.

4. Hydration
- **Importance:** Staying hydrated helps the kidneys flush out excess sugar through urine. Dehydration can lead to higher blood sugar levels.
- **Recommendation:** Aim to drink at least eight glasses of water a day.

5. Stress Management
- **Impact:** Stress can raise blood sugar levels due to the release of stress hormones like cortisol.
- **Techniques:** Practice stress-reducing activities such as yoga, meditation, deep breathing exercises, and hobbies that promote relaxation.

6. Medication Adherence
- **Importance:** Take medications as prescribed by your healthcare provider. Skipping doses or not following the prescribed regimen can lead to uncontrolled blood sugar levels.
- **Review:** Regularly review your medications with your healthcare provider to ensure they are still effective and appropriate for your needs.

Understanding Complications and Preventive Measures

Diabetes can lead to several complications if not managed properly. Understanding these complications and taking preventive measures is crucial for maintaining long-term health.

1. Cardiovascular Disease
- **Risk:** High blood sugar levels can damage blood vessels and increase the risk of heart disease and stroke.

- **Prevention:** Maintain a heart-healthy diet, exercise regularly, manage blood pressure and cholesterol levels, and avoid smoking.

2. **Neuropathy**
- **Risk:** Nerve damage, particularly in the legs and feet, can result from prolonged high blood sugar levels.
- **Prevention:** Keep blood sugar levels within the target range, practice good foot care, and get regular check-ups.

3. **Retinopathy**
- **Risk:** High blood sugar levels can damage the blood vessels in the eyes, leading to vision problems or blindness.
- **Prevention:** Regular eye exams, maintaining blood sugar control, and managing blood pressure.

4. **Kidney Disease**
- **Risk:** Diabetes can damage the kidneys over time, leading to chronic kidney disease or kidney failure.
- **Prevention:** Monitor kidney function, maintain blood sugar and blood pressure levels, and avoid excessive protein intake.

5. **Foot Problems**
- **Risk:** Poor circulation and nerve damage can lead to foot ulcers and infections.
- **Prevention:** Inspect feet daily, wear comfortable shoes, and seek prompt medical attention for any sores or infections.

Conclusion

Understanding diabetes and its impact on your body is the first step towards effective management. By comprehending the roles of different types of foods, the importance of the glycemic index, and the strategies for maintaining balanced blood sugar levels, you can take control of your health. Combining a diabetes-friendly diet with air frying offers a delicious, healthy way to manage your condition. The insights provided in this chapter, combined with the delicious and diabetes-friendly recipes in this cookbook, will help you lead a healthier and more fulfilling life. Embrace the knowledge, make informed choices, and enjoy the journey towards better diabetes management and overall well-being.

Chapter 3

Breakfast Recipes

① Air-Fried Veggie Omelette Cups 18

② Cinnamon Apple Breakfast Bites 18

③ Spinach and Feta Egg Muffins.......................................19

④ Berry Almond Breakfast Squares 19

⑤ Greek Yogurt Parfait with Air-Fried Granola 20

⑥ Avocado and Egg Breakfast Boats..................................20

⑦ Banana Walnut Morning Muffins 21

⑧ Zucchini and Cheese Frittata Slices 21

⑨ Blueberry Lemon Ricotta Pancake Bites.........................22

⑩ Breakfast Stuffed Bell Peppers......................................22

⑪ Air-Fried Breakfast Burrito Bowl...................................23

⑫ Spinach and Mushroom Egg Cups 23

⑬ Peanut Butter Banana Breakfast Roll-Ups 24

⑭ Mediterranean Breakfast Pita Pockets...........................24

⑮ Apple Cinnamon French Toast Sticks.............................25

⑯ Egg and Turkey Bacon Breakfast Tacos 25

⑰ Quinoa and Berry Breakfast Bowl..................................26

⑱ Air-Fried Breakfast Sausage Patties...............................26

⑲ Veggie-Packed Breakfast Casserole Cups 27

⑳ Protein-Packed Breakfast Sandwiches............................27

Chapter 3: Breakfast Recipes

1. Air-Fried Veggie Omelette Cups

Ingredients:
- 1 cup spinach, chopped
- 1/2 cup bell peppers, diced
- 1/2 cup mushrooms, sliced
- 6 large eggs
- 1/4 cup skim milk
- 1/4 cup shredded low-fat cheddar cheese
- Salt and pepper to taste
- Cooking spray

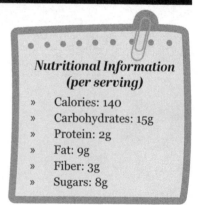

Nutritional Information (per serving)
- » Calories: 110
- » Carbohydrates: 3g
- » Protein: 9g
- » Fat: 7g
- » Fiber: 1g
- » Sugars: 2g

Instructions:
1. Preheat your air fryer to 350°F.
2. In a large bowl, whisk together the eggs, skim milk, salt, and pepper.
3. Spray silicone muffin cups with cooking spray and place them in the air fryer basket.
4. Divide the chopped spinach, diced bell peppers, and sliced mushrooms evenly among the muffin cups.
5. Pour the egg mixture into each cup, filling them about 3/4 full.
6. Sprinkle shredded cheddar cheese on top of each cup.
7. Cook in the air fryer for 10-12 minutes or until the omelette cups are set and slightly golden.
8. Carefully remove the muffin cups from the air fryer and let them cool slightly before serving.

2. Cinnamon Apple Breakfast Bites

Ingredients:
- 2 large apples, peeled, cored, and diced
- 1 tsp ground cinnamon
- 1 tbsp stevia or other sugar substitute
- 1/4 cup almond flour
- 1/4 cup rolled oats
- 1/4 cup chopped walnuts
- 1 tbsp melted coconut oil

Nutritional Information (per serving)
- » Calories: 140
- » Carbohydrates: 15g
- » Protein: 2g
- » Fat: 9g
- » Fiber: 3g
- » Sugars: 8g

Instructions:
1. Preheat your air fryer to 360°F.
2. In a bowl, combine the diced apples, ground cinnamon, and stevia.
3. In another bowl, mix together the almond flour, rolled oats, chopped walnuts, and melted coconut oil.
4. Spray a small baking dish with cooking spray and add the apple mixture, spreading it evenly.
5. Sprinkle the almond flour mixture over the apples.
6. Place the baking dish in the air fryer and cook for 15-20 minutes until the topping is golden brown and the apples are tender.
7. Let it cool for a few minutes before serving.

3. Spinach and Feta Egg Muffins

Ingredients:
- 1 cup fresh spinach, chopped
- 1/4 cup feta cheese, crumbled
- 6 large eggs
- 1/4 cup skim milk
- 1/2 tsp garlic powder
- Salt and pepper to taste
- Cooking spray

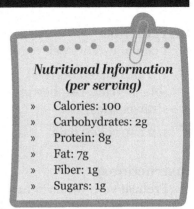

Nutritional Information (per serving)
- » Calories: 100
- » Carbohydrates: 2g
- » Protein: 8g
- » Fat: 7g
- » Fiber: 1g
- » Sugars: 1g

Instructions:
1. Preheat your air fryer to 350°F.
2. In a large bowl, whisk together the eggs, skim milk, garlic powder, salt, and pepper.
3. Spray silicone muffin cups with cooking spray and place them in the air fryer basket.
4. Divide the chopped spinach and crumbled feta cheese evenly among the muffin cups.
5. Pour the egg mixture into each cup, filling them about 3/4 full.
6. Cook in the air fryer for 10-12 minutes or until the egg muffins are set and slightly golden.
7. Carefully remove the muffin cups from the air fryer and let them cool slightly before serving.

4. Berry Almond Breakfast Squares

Ingredients:
- 1 cup rolled oats
- 1/2 cup almond flour
- 1/4 cup stevia or other sugar substitute
- 1 tsp baking powder
- 1/2 tsp ground cinnamon
- 1/4 cup unsweetened applesauce
- 1/4 cup almond milk
- 1 large egg
- 1 tsp vanilla extract
- 1 cup mixed berries (blueberries, raspberries, strawberries)
- 1/4 cup sliced almonds

Nutritional Information (per serving)
- » Calories: 150
- » Carbohydrates: 18g
- » Protein: 4g
- » Fat: 7g
- » Fiber: 3g
- » Sugars: 5g

Instructions:
1. Preheat your air fryer to 350°F.
2. In a large bowl, combine the rolled oats, almond flour, stevia, baking powder, and ground cinnamon.
3. In another bowl, mix together the unsweetened applesauce, almond milk, egg, and vanilla extract.
4. Add the wet ingredients to the dry ingredients and stir until well combined.
5. Gently fold in the mixed berries.
6. Line a small baking dish with parchment paper and pour the batter into the dish, spreading it evenly.
7. Sprinkle the sliced almonds on top.
8. Place the baking dish in the air fryer and cook for 20-25 minutes until the top is golden brown and a toothpick inserted into the center comes out clean.
9. Let it cool before cutting into squares and serving.

5. Greek Yogurt Parfait with Air-Fried Granola

Ingredients:
- 1 cup non-fat Greek yogurt
- 1/2 cup mixed berries (blueberries, raspberries, strawberries)
- 1/2 cup rolled oats
- 2 tbsp chopped nuts (almonds, walnuts, or pecans)
- 1 tbsp melted coconut oil
- 1 tbsp honey or sugar-free syrup
- 1/2 tsp ground cinnamon

Nutritional Information (per serving)
- » Calories: 220
- » Carbohydrates: 30g
- » Protein: 10g
- » Fat: 8g
- » Fiber: 4g
- » Sugars: 12g

Instructions:
1. Preheat your air fryer to 300°F.
2. In a bowl, mix together the rolled oats, chopped nuts, melted coconut oil, honey, and ground cinnamon until well coated.
3. Spread the oat mixture evenly in the air fryer basket lined with parchment paper.
4. Cook in the air fryer for 10-12 minutes, shaking the basket halfway through, until the granola is golden and crispy.
5. In a serving glass or bowl, layer the Greek yogurt, mixed berries, and air-fried granola.
6. Serve immediately.

6. Avocado and Egg Breakfast Boats

Ingredients:
- 2 large avocados
- 4 large eggs
- Salt and pepper to taste
- 1/4 cup shredded low-fat cheddar cheese
- 1 tbsp chopped fresh chives (optional)
- Cooking spray

Nutritional Information (per serving)
- » Calories: 280
- » Carbohydrates: 10g
- » Protein: 12g
- » Fat: 23g
- » Fiber: 7g
- » Sugars: 1g

Instructions:
1. Preheat your air fryer to 350°F.
2. Cut the avocados in half and remove the pits. Scoop out a small amount of avocado flesh to create enough space for the eggs.
3. Place the avocado halves in the air fryer basket, making sure they are stable. Use aluminum foil to create a nest if needed to keep them upright.
4. Crack an egg into each avocado half, season with salt and pepper, and sprinkle with shredded cheddar cheese.
5. Cook in the air fryer for 12-15 minutes or until the eggs are cooked to your desired doneness.
6. Sprinkle with chopped fresh chives before serving, if desired.

7. Banana Walnut Morning Muffins

Ingredients:
- 1 cup whole wheat flour
- 1/2 cup almond flour
- 1/4 cup stevia or other sugar substitute
- 1 tsp baking soda
- 1/2 tsp ground cinnamon
- 1/4 tsp salt
- 2 ripe bananas, mashed
- 1/4 cup unsweetened applesauce
- 1/4 cup almond milk
- 2 large eggs
- 1 tsp vanilla extract
- 1/2 cup chopped walnuts

Nutritional Information (per serving)
- » Calories: 180
- » Carbohydrates: 24g
- » Protein: 6g
- » Fat: 8g
- » Fiber: 4g
- » Sugars: 7g

Instructions:
1. Preheat your air fryer to 320°F.
2. In a large bowl, combine the whole wheat flour, almond flour, stevia, baking soda, ground cinnamon, and salt.
3. In another bowl, mix together the mashed bananas, unsweetened applesauce, almond milk, eggs, and vanilla extract.
4. Add the wet ingredients to the dry ingredients and stir until just combined.
5. Fold in the chopped walnuts.
6. Spray silicone muffin cups with cooking spray and fill them with the batter.
7. Place the muffin cups in the air fryer basket and cook for 12-15 minutes, or until a toothpick inserted into the center comes out clean.
8. Allow the muffins to cool slightly before removing them from the cups and serving.

8. Zucchini and Cheese Frittata Slices

Ingredients:
- 1 medium zucchini, grated
- 1/4 cup grated Parmesan cheese
- 1/4 cup shredded low-fat mozzarella cheese
- 6 large eggs
- 1/4 cup skim milk
- 1/2 tsp garlic powder
- 1/2 tsp dried oregano
- Salt and pepper to taste
- Cooking spray

Nutritional Information (per serving)
- » Calories: 120
- » Carbohydrates: 3g
- » Protein: 10g
- » Fat: 7g
- » Fiber: 1g
- » Sugars: 1g

Instructions:
1. Preheat your air fryer to 350°F.
2. In a large bowl, whisk together the eggs, skim milk, garlic powder, dried oregano, salt, and pepper.
3. Stir in the grated zucchini, Parmesan cheese, and mozzarella cheese.
4. Spray a small baking dish with cooking spray and pour the mixture into the dish.
5. Place the dish in the air fryer and cook for 12-15 minutes or until the frittata is set and golden brown.
6. Allow to cool slightly before slicing and serving.

9. Blueberry Lemon Ricotta Pancake Bites

Ingredients:
- 1 cup ricotta cheese
- 2 large eggs
- 1/4 cup almond flour
- 1/2 tsp baking powder
- 1/2 tsp vanilla extract
- Zest of 1 lemon
- 1/2 cup fresh blueberries
- Cooking spray

Nutritional Information (per serving)
- » Calories: 90
- » Carbohydrates: 6g
- » Protein: 6g
- » Fat: 5g
- » Fiber: 1g
- » Sugars: 3g

Instructions:
1. Preheat your air fryer to 320°F.
2. In a large bowl, mix together the ricotta cheese, eggs, almond flour, baking powder, vanilla extract, and lemon zest until smooth.
3. Gently fold in the fresh blueberries.
4. Spray silicone muffin cups with cooking spray and fill them with the batter.
5. Place the muffin cups in the air fryer basket and cook for 12-15 minutes, or until the pancake bites are set and golden brown.
6. Allow to cool slightly before removing them from the cups and serving.

10. Breakfast Stuffed Bell Peppers

Ingredients:
- 2 large bell peppers, halved and seeds removed
- 4 large eggs
- 1/4 cup chopped spinach
- 1/4 cup diced tomatoes
- 1/4 cup shredded low-fat cheddar cheese
- Salt and pepper to taste
- Cooking spray

Nutritional Information (per serving)
- » Calories: 140
- » Carbohydrates: 7g
- » Protein: 10g
- » Fat: 9g
- » Fiber: 2g
- » Sugars: 3g

Instructions:
1. Preheat your air fryer to 350°F.
2. Spray the inside of the bell pepper halves with cooking spray and place them in the air fryer basket.
3. In a bowl, whisk together the eggs, chopped spinach, diced tomatoes, salt, and pepper.
4. Pour the egg mixture into the bell pepper halves, filling them about 3/4 full.
5. Sprinkle shredded cheddar cheese on top.
6. Cook in the air fryer for 12-15 minutes or until the eggs are set and the bell peppers are tender.
7. Allow to cool slightly before serving.

11. Air-Fried Breakfast Burrito Bowl

Ingredients:

- 1/2 cup cooked quinoa
- 1/2 cup black beans, drained and rinsed
- 1/4 cup diced bell peppers
- 1/4 cup diced onions
- 1/4 cup chopped tomatoes
- 1/4 cup shredded low-fat cheddar cheese
- 2 large eggs
- 1/4 tsp cumin
- 1/4 tsp paprika
- Salt and pepper to taste
- Cooking spray

Nutritional Information (per serving)

- » Calories: 250
- » Carbohydrates: 30g
- » Protein: 14g
- » Fat: 10g
- » Fiber: 6g
- » Sugars: 3g

Instructions:

1. Preheat your air fryer to 350°F.
2. In a bowl, mix together the cooked quinoa, black beans, diced bell peppers, diced onions, chopped tomatoes, cumin, paprika, salt, and pepper.
3. Spray a small baking dish with cooking spray and spread the quinoa mixture evenly in the dish.
4. Crack the eggs on top of the quinoa mixture.
5. Sprinkle shredded cheddar cheese over the eggs.
6. Place the baking dish in the air fryer and cook for 12-15 minutes or until the eggs are set and the cheese is melted.
7. Allow to cool slightly before serving.

12. Spinach and Mushroom Egg Cups

Ingredients:

- 1 cup chopped spinach
- 1/2 cup sliced mushrooms
- 6 large eggs
- 1/4 cup skim milk
- 1/4 cup shredded low-fat mozzarella cheese
- Salt and pepper to taste
- Cooking spray

Nutritional Information (per serving)

- » Calories: 100
- » Carbohydrates: 2g
- » Protein: 10g
- » Fat: 6g
- » Fiber: 1g
- » Sugars: 1g

Instructions:

1. Preheat your air fryer to 350°F.
2. In a large bowl, whisk together the eggs, skim milk, salt, and pepper.
3. Spray silicone muffin cups with cooking spray and place them in the air fryer basket.
4. Divide the chopped spinach and sliced mushrooms evenly among the muffin cups.
5. Pour the egg mixture into each cup, filling them about 3/4 full.
6. Sprinkle shredded mozzarella cheese on top of each cup.
7. Cook in the air fryer for 10-12 minutes or until the egg cups are set and slightly golden.
8. Carefully remove the muffin cups from the air fryer and let them cool slightly before serving.

13. Peanut Butter Banana Breakfast Roll-Ups

Ingredients:
- 2 whole wheat tortillas
- 2 tbsp natural peanut butter
- 1 large banana, sliced
- 1 tsp ground cinnamon
- Cooking spray

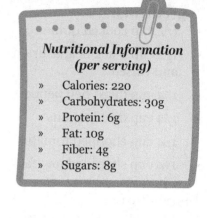

Nutritional Information (per serving)
- » Calories: 220
- » Carbohydrates: 30g
- » Protein: 6g
- » Fat: 10g
- » Fiber: 4g
- » Sugars: 8g

Instructions:
1. Preheat your air fryer to 350°F.
2. Spread 1 tablespoon of peanut butter on each whole wheat tortilla.
3. Place the banana slices on top of the peanut butter, then sprinkle with ground cinnamon.
4. Roll up the tortillas tightly and secure with toothpicks if needed.
5. Spray the roll-ups lightly with cooking spray.
6. Place the roll-ups in the air fryer basket and cook for 5-7 minutes or until the tortillas are crispy and golden.
7. Allow to cool slightly before serving.

14. Mediterranean Breakfast Pita Pockets

Ingredients:
- 2 whole wheat pita pockets
- 1/2 cup hummus
- 1/2 cup diced cucumber
- 1/2 cup diced tomatoes
- 1/4 cup crumbled feta cheese
- 1/4 cup chopped fresh parsley
- 2 large hard-boiled eggs, sliced
- Salt and pepper to taste

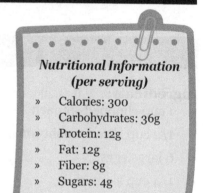

Nutritional Information (per serving)
- » Calories: 300
- » Carbohydrates: 36g
- » Protein: 12g
- » Fat: 12g
- » Fiber: 8g
- » Sugars: 4g

Instructions:
1. Preheat your air fryer to 350°F.
2. Cut the pita pockets in half and gently open them to create pockets.
3. Spread hummus inside each pita half.
4. Fill the pita pockets with diced cucumber, diced tomatoes, crumbled feta cheese, and sliced hard-boiled eggs.
5. Season with salt and pepper, and sprinkle with chopped fresh parsley.
6. Place the filled pita pockets in the air fryer basket and cook for 5-7 minutes or until the pitas are warm and slightly crispy.
7. Serve immediately.

15. Apple Cinnamon French Toast Sticks

Ingredients:
- 4 slices whole grain bread, cut into sticks
- 2 large eggs
- 1/4 cup unsweetened almond milk
- 1 tsp vanilla extract
- 1 tsp ground cinnamon
- 1 medium apple, peeled and finely diced
- Cooking spray

Nutritional Information (per serving)
- » Calories: 220
- » Carbohydrates: 32g
- » Protein: 9g
- » Fat: 6g
- » Fiber: 6g
- » Sugars: 10g

Instructions:
1. Preheat your air fryer to 350°F.
2. In a shallow bowl, whisk together the eggs, almond milk, vanilla extract, and ground cinnamon.
3. Dip the bread sticks into the egg mixture, ensuring they are well coated.
4. Spray the air fryer basket with cooking spray and place the coated bread sticks in a single layer in the basket.
5. Sprinkle the diced apple evenly over the bread sticks.
6. Cook in the air fryer for 8-10 minutes or until the bread sticks are golden brown and crispy.
7. Allow to cool slightly before serving.

16. Egg and Turkey Bacon Breakfast Tacos

Ingredients:
- 4 small corn tortillas
- 4 large eggs
- 1/4 cup skim milk
- 4 slices turkey bacon, cooked and crumbled
- 1/4 cup diced tomatoes
- 1/4 cup shredded low-fat cheddar cheese
- 1 tbsp chopped fresh cilantro
- Salt and pepper to taste
- Cooking spray

Nutritional Information (per serving)
- » Calories: 180
- » Carbohydrates: 14g
- » Protein: 14g
- » Fat: 8g
- » Fiber: 2g
- » Sugars: 2g

Instructions:
1. Preheat your air fryer to 350°F.
2. In a bowl, whisk together the eggs, skim milk, salt, and pepper.
3. Spray a small non-stick skillet with cooking spray and scramble the eggs over medium heat until fully cooked.
4. Warm the corn tortillas in the air fryer for 1-2 minutes.
5. Divide the scrambled eggs among the tortillas.
6. Top each taco with crumbled turkey bacon, diced tomatoes, shredded cheddar cheese, and chopped cilantro.
7. Serve immediately.

17. Quinoa and Berry Breakfast Bowl

Ingredients:
- 1/2 cup cooked quinoa
- 1/4 cup fresh blueberries
- 1/4 cup fresh raspberries
- 1/4 cup fresh strawberries, sliced
- 1/4 cup unsweetened almond milk
- 1 tbsp chopped almonds
- 1 tbsp chia seeds
- 1 tsp ground cinnamon

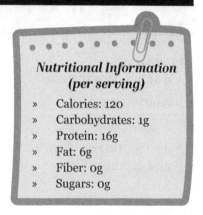

Nutritional Information (per serving)
- » Calories: 220
- » Carbohydrates: 35g
- » Protein: 7g
- » Fat: 7g
- » Fiber: 8g
- » Sugars: 8g

Instructions:
1. In a bowl, combine the cooked quinoa, blueberries, raspberries, and strawberries.
2. Pour the almond milk over the quinoa and berries.
3. Top with chopped almonds, chia seeds, and ground cinnamon.
4. Serve immediately.

18. Air-Fried Breakfast Sausage Patties

Ingredients:
- 1 lb ground turkey
- 1 tsp garlic powder
- 1 tsp onion powder
- 1 tsp dried sage
- 1/2 tsp dried thyme
- 1/2 tsp black pepper
- 1/2 tsp salt
- 1/4 tsp crushed red pepper flakes (optional)
- Cooking spray

Nutritional Information (per serving)
- » Calories: 120
- » Carbohydrates: 1g
- » Protein: 16g
- » Fat: 6g
- » Fiber: 0g
- » Sugars: 0g

Instructions:
1. Preheat your air fryer to 370°F.
2. In a large bowl, combine the ground turkey, garlic powder, onion powder, dried sage, dried thyme, black pepper, salt, and crushed red pepper flakes.
3. Form the mixture into small patties, about 2 inches in diameter.
4. Spray the air fryer basket with cooking spray and place the patties in a single layer in the basket.
5. Cook in the air fryer for 10-12 minutes, flipping halfway through, until the patties are golden brown and cooked through.
6. Allow to cool slightly before serving.

19. Veggie-Packed Breakfast Casserole Cups

Ingredients:
- 1/2 cup diced bell peppers
- 1/2 cup chopped spinach
- 1/4 cup diced onions
- 6 large eggs
- 1/4 cup skim milk
- 1/4 cup shredded low-fat mozzarella cheese
- Salt and pepper to taste
- Cooking spray

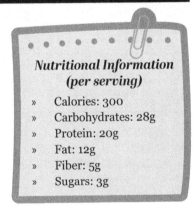

Nutritional Information (per serving)
» Calories: 90
» Carbohydrates: 3g
» Protein: 9g
» Fat: 5g
» Fiber: 1g
» Sugars: 1g

Instructions:
1. Preheat your air fryer to 350°F.
2. In a large bowl, whisk together the eggs, skim milk, salt, and pepper.
3. Spray silicone muffin cups with cooking spray and place them in the air fryer basket.
4. Divide the diced bell peppers, chopped spinach, and diced onions evenly among the muffin cups.
5. Pour the egg mixture into each cup, filling them about 3/4 full.
6. Sprinkle shredded mozzarella cheese on top of each cup.
7. Cook in the air fryer for 10-12 minutes or until the casserole cups are set and slightly golden.
8. Carefully remove the muffin cups from the air fryer and let them cool slightly before serving.

20. Protein-Packed Breakfast Sandwiches

Ingredients:
- 4 whole grain English muffins, split and toasted
- 4 large eggs
- 4 slices turkey bacon, cooked
- 1/4 cup guacamole
- 4 slices tomato
- 1/4 cup baby spinach
- Salt and pepper to taste
- Cooking spray

Nutritional Information (per serving)
» Calories: 300
» Carbohydrates: 28g
» Protein: 20g
» Fat: 12g
» Fiber: 5g
» Sugars: 3g

Instructions:
1. Preheat your air fryer to 350°F.
2. Spray a small non-stick skillet with cooking spray and cook the eggs over medium heat until the whites are set but the yolks are still slightly runny. Season with salt and pepper.
3. Spread 1 tablespoon of guacamole on each English muffin half.
4. Assemble the sandwiches by layering the cooked eggs, turkey bacon, tomato slices, and baby spinach on the bottom halves of the English muffins.
5. Top with the other half of the English muffin.
6. Place the assembled sandwiches in the air fryer basket and cook for 3-5 minutes until the sandwiches are warm and the muffins are crispy.
7. Serve immediately.

These breakfast recipes are tailored to be healthy and suitable for individuals managing diabetes, while utilizing the convenience and benefits of air frying. Enjoy these delicious and nutritious meals to start your day on the right note!

Chapter 4

Morning Snack Recipes

1 Crunchy Cucumber Dippers with Hummus 29

2 Almond Butter Banana Bites..................................29

3 Greek Yogurt Blueberry Bark................................30

4 Crispy Parmesan Zucchini Chips 30

5 Spiced Pumpkin Seed Clusters..............................31

6 Mini Bell Pepper Poppers with Cream Cheese 31

7 Coconut Almond Energy Bites 32

8 Air-Fried Cinnamon Pear Slices............................32

9 Turkey Jerky and Cheese Stacks 33

10 Chocolate Covered Raspberry Clusters....................33

11 Tomato Basil Mozzarella Skewers..........................34

12 Coconut Lime Energy Balls 34

13 Honey Mustard Roasted Chickpeas 35

14 Apple Pie Trail Mix.......................................35

15 Crunchy Broccoli Cauliflower Bites.......................36

16 Cranberry Orange Almond Bars.............................36

17 Tangy Pickle Snack Sticks 37

18 Lemon Garlic Edamame Pods................................37

19 Sweet and Spicy Pecan Halves 38

20 Roasted Beetroot Chips with Sea Salt.....................38

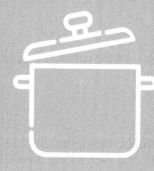

Chapter 4: Morning Snack Recipes

1. Crunchy Cucumber Dippers with Hummus

Ingredients:
- 2 large cucumbers
- 1 cup store-bought hummus
- 1 tsp garlic powder
- 1 tsp paprika
- 1 tbsp olive oil
- Salt to taste

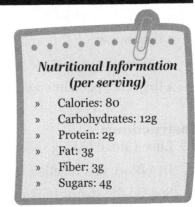

Nutritional Information (per serving)
- » Calories: 80
- » Carbohydrates: 12g
- » Protein: 2g
- » Fat: 3g
- » Fiber: 3g
- » Sugars: 4g

Instructions:
1. Preheat your air fryer to 350°F.
2. Peel the cucumbers and cut them into sticks.
3. In a bowl, toss the cucumber sticks with olive oil, garlic powder, paprika, and salt.
4. Place the cucumber sticks in the air fryer basket in a single layer.
5. Air fry for 10-12 minutes or until they are crispy and golden.
6. Serve with store-bought hummus for dipping.

2. Almond Butter Banana Bites

Ingredients:
- 2 large bananas
- 1/4 cup natural almond butter
- 1 tbsp chia seeds
- 1 tsp cinnamon
- Cooking spray

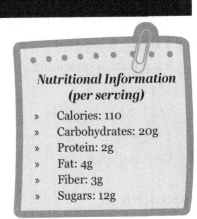

Nutritional Information (per serving)
- » Calories: 110
- » Carbohydrates: 20g
- » Protein: 2g
- » Fat: 4g
- » Fiber: 3g
- » Sugars: 12g

Instructions:
1. Preheat your air fryer to 350°F.
2. Slice the bananas into 1-inch thick rounds.
3. Spread a small amount of almond butter on each banana slice.
4. Sprinkle chia seeds and a pinch of cinnamon on top of the almond butter.
5. Lightly spray the air fryer basket with cooking spray and place the banana slices in a single layer.
6. Air fry for 5-7 minutes or until the bananas are warm and the almond butter is slightly melted.
7. Serve immediately.

3. Greek Yogurt Blueberry Bark

Ingredients:
- 1 cup non-fat Greek yogurt
- 1/2 cup fresh blueberries
- 1 tbsp honey
- 1 tsp vanilla extract
- 1 tbsp chopped almonds

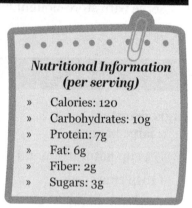

Nutritional Information (per serving)
- » Calories: 90
- » Carbohydrates: 12g
- » Protein: 6g
- » Fat: 3g
- » Fiber: 1g
- » Sugars: 9g

Instructions:
1. Line a small baking sheet with parchment paper.
2. In a bowl, mix together the Greek yogurt, honey, and vanilla extract.
3. Spread the yogurt mixture evenly on the parchment paper.
4. Sprinkle the fresh blueberries and chopped almonds over the yogurt.
5. Freeze for at least 2 hours or until the yogurt is firm.
6. Break into pieces and serve immediately.

4. Crispy Parmesan Zucchini Chips

Ingredients:
- 2 medium zucchinis
- 1/2 cup grated Parmesan cheese
- 1/2 cup whole wheat breadcrumbs
- 1 tsp garlic powder
- 1 tsp Italian seasoning
- 1/4 tsp salt
- 1/4 tsp black pepper
- 1 large egg
- Cooking spray

Nutritional Information (per serving)
- » Calories: 120
- » Carbohydrates: 10g
- » Protein: 7g
- » Fat: 6g
- » Fiber: 2g
- » Sugars: 3g

Instructions:
1. Preheat your air fryer to 400°F.
2. Slice the zucchinis into thin rounds.
3. In a bowl, mix together the grated Parmesan cheese, whole wheat breadcrumbs, garlic powder, Italian seasoning, salt, and black pepper.
4. In another bowl, beat the egg.
5. Dip each zucchini slice into the egg, then coat with the breadcrumb mixture.
6. Spray the air fryer basket with cooking spray and place the zucchini slices in a single layer.
7. Air fry for 10-12 minutes or until the zucchini chips are golden brown and crispy.
8. Serve immediately.

5. Spiced Pumpkin Seed Clusters

Ingredients:
- 1 cup raw pumpkin seeds
- 1 tbsp olive oil
- 1 tsp cinnamon
- 1/2 tsp ground ginger
- 1/2 tsp ground nutmeg
- 1/4 tsp salt
- 1 tbsp honey

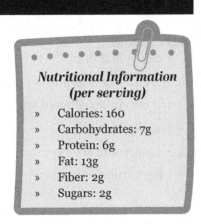

Nutritional Information (per serving)
- » Calories: 160
- » Carbohydrates: 7g
- » Protein: 6g
- » Fat: 13g
- » Fiber: 2g
- » Sugars: 2g

Instructions:
1. Preheat your air fryer to 350°F.
2. In a bowl, mix together the pumpkin seeds, olive oil, cinnamon, ground ginger, ground nutmeg, salt, and honey until the seeds are well coated.
3. Spread the pumpkin seeds evenly in the air fryer basket.
4. Air fry for 10-12 minutes, shaking the basket halfway through, until the seeds are golden and crispy.
5. Let cool completely before serving.

6. Mini Bell Pepper Poppers with Cream Cheese

Ingredients:
- 8 mini bell peppers
- 4 oz low-fat cream cheese
- 1/4 cup shredded low-fat cheddar cheese
- 1 tsp garlic powder
- 1/2 tsp paprika
- Salt and pepper to taste
- Cooking spray

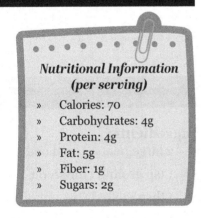

Nutritional Information (per serving)
- » Calories: 70
- » Carbohydrates: 4g
- » Protein: 4g
- » Fat: 5g
- » Fiber: 1g
- » Sugars: 2g

Instructions:
1. Preheat your air fryer to 370°F.
2. Cut the mini bell peppers in half and remove the seeds.
3. In a bowl, mix together the low-fat cream cheese, shredded cheddar cheese, garlic powder, paprika, salt, and pepper until smooth.
4. Fill each bell pepper half with the cream cheese mixture.
5. Spray the air fryer basket with cooking spray and place the stuffed bell peppers in a single layer.
6. Air fry for 8-10 minutes or until the peppers are tender and the cheese is melted and golden.
7. Serve immediately.

7. Coconut Almond Energy Bites

Ingredients:
- 1 cup rolled oats
- 1/2 cup almond butter
- 1/4 cup unsweetened shredded coconut
- 1/4 cup honey
- 1/4 cup chia seeds
- 1 tsp vanilla extract

Nutritional Information (per serving)
- » Calories: 110
- » Carbohydrates: 12g
- » Protein: 3g
- » Fat: 6g
- » Fiber: 3g
- » Sugars: 6g

Instructions:
1. In a large bowl, mix together the rolled oats, almond butter, shredded coconut, honey, chia seeds, and vanilla extract until well combined.
2. Roll the mixture into small balls, about 1 inch in diameter.
3. Place the energy bites in the air fryer basket in a single layer.
4. Air fry at 350°F for 5-7 minutes or until they are lightly browned.
5. Let cool completely before serving.

8. Air-Fried Cinnamon Pear Slices

Ingredients:
- 2 large pears, cored and sliced
- 1 tsp ground cinnamon
- 1 tbsp melted coconut oil
- 1 tbsp honey

Nutritional Information (per serving)
- » Calories: 90
- » Carbohydrates: 22g
- » Protein: 1g
- » Fat: 3g
- » Fiber: 4g
- » Sugars: 16g

Instructions:
1. Preheat your air fryer to 350°F.
2. In a bowl, toss the pear slices with melted coconut oil, ground cinnamon, and honey until well coated.
3. Place the pear slices in the air fryer basket in a single layer.
4. Air fry for 8-10 minutes or until the pears are tender and slightly caramelized.
5. Serve immediately.

9. Turkey Jerky and Cheese Stacks

Ingredients:
- 8 oz turkey breast, sliced thin
- 1/2 cup low-fat cheddar cheese, sliced into small squares
- 1 tsp garlic powder
- 1 tsp onion powder
- 1/2 tsp smoked paprika
- 1/4 tsp salt
- Cooking spray

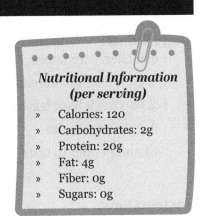

Nutritional Information (per serving)
- » Calories: 120
- » Carbohydrates: 2g
- » Protein: 20g
- » Fat: 4g
- » Fiber: 0g
- » Sugars: 0g

Instructions:
1. Preheat your air fryer to 200°F.
2. In a bowl, mix together the garlic powder, onion powder, smoked paprika, and salt.
3. Rub the spice mixture onto the turkey breast slices.
4. Lightly spray the air fryer basket with cooking spray and arrange the turkey slices in a single layer.
5. Air fry for 2-3 hours, flipping halfway through, until the turkey is dry and chewy.
6. Let cool and stack with cheese squares to serve.

10. Chocolate Covered Raspberry Clusters

Ingredients:
- 1 cup fresh raspberries
- 1/2 cup dark chocolate chips
- 1 tsp coconut oil

Nutritional Information (per serving)
- » Calories: 100
- » Carbohydrates: 14g
- » Protein: 1g
- » Fat: 6g
- » Fiber: 4g
- » Sugars: 8g

Instructions:
1. Line a small baking sheet with parchment paper.
2. In a microwave-safe bowl, melt the dark chocolate chips and coconut oil together, stirring until smooth.
3. Dip each raspberry into the melted chocolate and place it on the parchment paper.
4. Freeze for at least 30 minutes or until the chocolate is set.
5. Serve immediately or store in the freezer for a quick snack.

11. Tomato Basil Mozzarella Skewers

Ingredients:
- 1 cup cherry tomatoes
- 1/2 cup fresh mozzarella balls
- 1/4 cup fresh basil leaves
- 1 tbsp balsamic glaze
- Salt and pepper to taste

Instructions:
1. Thread the cherry tomatoes, mozzarella balls, and basil leaves onto small skewers, alternating as you go.
2. Season with salt and pepper to taste.
3. Drizzle with balsamic glaze before serving.

Nutritional Information (per serving)
- » Calories: 80
- » Carbohydrates: 4g
- » Protein: 5g
- » Fat: 5g
- » Fiber: 1g
- » Sugars: 3g

12. Coconut Lime Energy Balls

Ingredients:
- 1 cup rolled oats
- 1/2 cup shredded unsweetened coconut
- 1/4 cup almond butter
- 1/4 cup honey
- Zest of 1 lime
- 1 tbsp lime juice

Instructions:
1. In a large bowl, mix together the rolled oats, shredded coconut, almond butter, honey, lime zest, and lime juice until well combined.
2. Roll the mixture into small balls, about 1 inch in diameter.
3. Place the energy balls in the air fryer basket in a single layer.
4. Air fry at 350°F for 5-7 minutes or until they are lightly browned.
5. Let cool completely before serving.

Nutritional Information (per serving)
- » Calories: 100
- » Carbohydrates: 14g
- » Protein: 2g
- » Fat: 4g
- » Fiber: 2g
- » Sugars: 8g

13. Honey Mustard Roasted Chickpeas

Ingredients:
- 1 can chickpeas (15 oz), drained and rinsed
- 1 tbsp olive oil
- 1 tbsp honey
- 1 tbsp Dijon mustard
- 1 tsp garlic powder
- 1/2 tsp smoked paprika
- Salt and pepper to taste

Nutritional Information (per serving)
- » Calories: 140
- » Carbohydrates: 22g
- » Protein: 6g
- » Fat: 4g
- » Fiber: 6g
- » Sugars: 4g

Instructions:
1. Preheat your air fryer to 400°F.
2. In a bowl, mix together the olive oil, honey, Dijon mustard, garlic powder, smoked paprika, salt, and pepper.
3. Add the chickpeas and toss until well coated.
4. Spread the chickpeas evenly in the air fryer basket.
5. Air fry for 15-20 minutes, shaking the basket halfway through, until the chickpeas are crispy and golden.
6. Let cool before serving.

14. Apple Pie Trail Mix

Ingredients:
- 1 cup dried apple slices
- 1/2 cup raw almonds
- 1/2 cup raw walnuts
- 1/4 cup unsweetened coconut flakes
- 1 tsp ground cinnamon
- 1/4 tsp ground nutmeg

Nutritional Information (per serving)
- » Calories: 180
- » Carbohydrates: 20g
- » Protein: 4g
- » Fat: 10g
- » Fiber: 4g
- » Sugars: 12g

Instructions:
1. In a large bowl, mix together the dried apple slices, raw almonds, raw walnuts, coconut flakes, ground cinnamon, and ground nutmeg until well combined.
2. Store in an airtight container and enjoy as a quick snack.

15. Crunchy Broccoli Cauliflower Bites

Ingredients:
- 1 cup broccoli florets
- 1 cup cauliflower florets
- 1/4 cup grated Parmesan cheese
- 1/4 cup whole wheat breadcrumbs
- 1 tsp garlic powder
- 1/2 tsp Italian seasoning
- 1/4 tsp salt
- 1/4 tsp black pepper
- 1 large egg
- Cooking spray

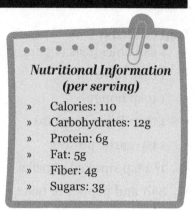

Nutritional Information (per serving)
- » Calories: 110
- » Carbohydrates: 12g
- » Protein: 6g
- » Fat: 5g
- » Fiber: 4g
- » Sugars: 3g

Instructions:
1. Preheat your air fryer to 400°F.
2. In a bowl, mix together the grated Parmesan cheese, whole wheat breadcrumbs, garlic powder, Italian seasoning, salt, and black pepper.
3. In another bowl, beat the egg.
4. Dip each broccoli and cauliflower floret into the egg, then coat with the breadcrumb mixture.
5. Spray the air fryer basket with cooking spray and place the florets in a single layer.
6. Air fry for 10-12 minutes or until the florets are golden brown and crispy.
7. Serve immediately.

16. Cranberry Orange Almond Bars

Ingredients:
- 1 cup rolled oats
- 1/2 cup almond flour
- 1/4 cup dried cranberries
- Zest of 1 orange
- 1/4 cup honey
- 1/4 cup almond butter
- 1 tsp vanilla extract

Nutritional Information (per serving)
- » Calories: 130
- » Carbohydrates: 18g
- » Protein: 3g
- » Fat: 6g
- » Fiber: 3g
- » Sugars: 10g

Instructions:
1. Preheat your air fryer to 350°F.
2. In a large bowl, mix together the rolled oats, almond flour, dried cranberries, orange zest, honey, almond butter, and vanilla extract until well combined.
3. Press the mixture into a small baking dish lined with parchment paper.
4. Air fry for 12-15 minutes or until the bars are set and lightly browned.
5. Let cool completely before cutting into bars and serving.

17. Tangy Pickle Snack Sticks

Ingredients:

- 2 large dill pickles
- 1/4 cup almond flour
- 1/4 cup grated Parmesan cheese
- 1 tsp garlic powder
- 1/2 tsp paprika
- 1/4 tsp black pepper
- 1 large egg
- Cooking spray

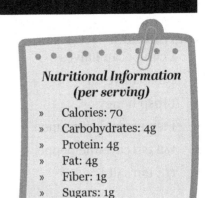

Nutritional Information (per serving)

» Calories: 70
» Carbohydrates: 4g
» Protein: 4g
» Fat: 4g
» Fiber: 1g
» Sugars: 1g

Instructions:

1. Preheat your air fryer to 400°F.
2. Cut the dill pickles into sticks.
3. In a bowl, mix together the almond flour, grated Parmesan cheese, garlic powder, paprika, and black pepper.
4. In another bowl, beat the egg.
5. Dip each pickle stick into the egg, then coat with the almond flour mixture.
6. Spray the air fryer basket with cooking spray and place the pickle sticks in a single layer.
7. Air fry for 8-10 minutes or until the pickle sticks are golden brown and crispy.
8. Serve immediately.

18. Lemon Garlic Edamame Pods

Ingredients:

- 2 cups edamame pods
- 1 tbsp olive oil
- 1 tsp garlic powder
- Zest of 1 lemon
- Salt to taste

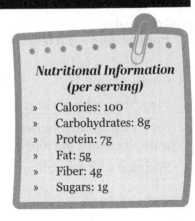

Nutritional Information (per serving)

» Calories: 100
» Carbohydrates: 8g
» Protein: 7g
» Fat: 5g
» Fiber: 4g
» Sugars: 1g

Instructions:

1. Preheat your air fryer to 375°F.
2. In a bowl, toss the edamame pods with olive oil, garlic powder, lemon zest, and salt.
3. Place the edamame pods in the air fryer basket in a single layer.
4. Air fry for 8-10 minutes or until the pods are crispy and slightly browned.
5. Serve immediately.

19. Sweet and Spicy Pecan Halves

Ingredients:
- 1 cup pecan halves
- 1 tbsp olive oil
- 1 tbsp honey
- 1 tsp ground cinnamon
- 1/2 tsp cayenne pepper
- 1/4 tsp salt

Nutritional Information (per serving)
- » Calories: 200
- » Carbohydrates: 10g
- » Protein: 2g
- » Fat: 19g
- » Fiber: 3g
- » Sugars: 6g

Instructions:
1. Preheat your air fryer to 350°F.
2. In a bowl, mix together the pecan halves, olive oil, honey, ground cinnamon, cayenne pepper, and salt until the pecans are well coated.
3. Spread the pecans evenly in the air fryer basket.
4. Air fry for 8-10 minutes, shaking the basket halfway through, until the pecans are golden and crispy.
5. Let cool completely before serving.

20. Roasted Beetroot Chips with Sea Salt

Ingredients:
- 2 large beetroots, peeled and thinly sliced
- 1 tbsp olive oil
- 1/2 tsp sea salt

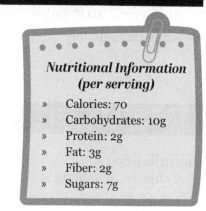

Nutritional Information (per serving)
- » Calories: 70
- » Carbohydrates: 10g
- » Protein: 2g
- » Fat: 3g
- » Fiber: 2g
- » Sugars: 7g

Instructions:
1. Preheat your air fryer to 350°F.
2. In a bowl, toss the beetroot slices with olive oil until they are evenly coated.
3. Place the beetroot slices in the air fryer basket in a single layer.
4. Air fry for 15-20 minutes, shaking the basket halfway through, until the beetroot chips are crispy.
5. Sprinkle with sea salt and let cool completely before serving.

These morning snack recipes are designed to be diabetic-friendly and easy to prepare using an air fryer, ensuring you get nutritious and delicious snacks to keep you energized throughout the day.

Chapter 5

Lunch Recipes

1. Air-Fried Chicken Caesar Salad Wraps...........................40

2. Greek Chicken Souvlaki Skewers with Tzatziki 41

3. Quinoa Stuffed Bell Peppers with Turkey......................42

4. BBQ Turkey Burger Sliders with Sweet Potato Fries......43

5. Southwest Black Bean and Corn Salad 43

6. Asian Sesame Ginger Tofu Salad 44

7. Mediterranean Veggie Wrap with Hummus...................44

8. Lemon Herb Grilled Shrimp Salad 45

9. Turkey and Avocado Lettuce Wraps 45

10. Caprese Panini with Balsamic Glaze.............................46

11. Air-Fried Falafel Pita Pockets with Tahini Sauce 46

12. Salmon Nicoise Salad with Dijon Dressing....................47

13. Rainbow Veggie Buddha Bowl with Quinoa 47

14. Air-Fried Coconut Shrimp Salad with Mango Salsa.......48

15. Buffalo Cauliflower Bites with Ranch Dip......................48

16. Greek Orzo Salad with Feta and Olives..........................49

17. Turkey and Cranberry Spinach Wrap 49

18. Shrimp and Mango Rice Paper Rolls 50

19. Lentil and Veggie Soup with Herbed Croutons 50

20. Hawaiian BBQ Chicken Salad Bowl 51

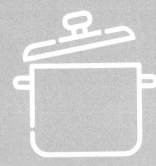

1. Air-Fried Chicken Caesar Salad Wraps

Ingredients:

- 2 boneless, skinless chicken breasts
- 1 tbsp olive oil
- 1 tsp garlic powder
- 1 tsp Italian seasoning
- 1/2 tsp salt
- 1/4 tsp black pepper
- 4 whole wheat tortillas
- 2 cups chopped romaine lettuce
- 1/2 cup shredded Parmesan cheese
- 1/2 cup Caesar dressing (low-fat or light)
- Cooking spray

Nutritional Information (per serving)

- » Calories: 300
- » Carbohydrates: 28g
- » Protein: 26g
- » Fat: 12g
- » Fiber: 4g
- » Sugars: 2g

Instructions:

1. Preheat your air fryer to 375°F.
2. In a bowl, mix the olive oil, garlic powder, Italian seasoning, salt, and black pepper. Coat the chicken breasts with this mixture.
3. Spray the air fryer basket with cooking spray and place the chicken breasts in a single layer.
4. Air fry for 15-20 minutes, flipping halfway through, until the chicken is cooked through and golden brown. Let it rest for 5 minutes before slicing.
5. Warm the whole wheat tortillas in the air fryer for 1-2 minutes.
6. Assemble the wraps by placing chopped romaine lettuce, sliced chicken, shredded Parmesan cheese, and Caesar dressing in each tortilla.
7. Roll up the tortillas and serve immediately.

Ingredients:

- 1 lb boneless, skinless chicken breasts, cut into 1-inch pieces
- 2 tbsp olive oil
- 2 tbsp lemon juice
- 2 cloves garlic, minced
- 1 tbsp dried oregano
- 1 tsp salt
- 1/2 tsp black pepper
- 1 cup diced cucumber
- 1 cup Greek yogurt (non-fat)
- 1 tbsp fresh dill, chopped
- 1 tbsp lemon juice
- 1 clove garlic, minced
- Salt and pepper to taste
- Wooden skewers, soaked in water for 30 minutes
- Cooking spray

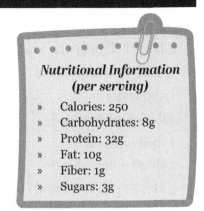

Nutritional Information (per serving)

» Calories: 250
» Carbohydrates: 8g
» Protein: 32g
» Fat: 10g
» Fiber: 1g
» Sugars: 3g

Instructions:

1. Preheat your air fryer to 375°F.
2. In a bowl, mix the olive oil, lemon juice, minced garlic, dried oregano, salt, and black pepper. Add the chicken pieces and marinate for at least 30 minutes.
3. Thread the marinated chicken onto the soaked wooden skewers.
4. Spray the air fryer basket with cooking spray and place the skewers in a single layer.
5. Air fry for 12-15 minutes, flipping halfway through, until the chicken is cooked through and slightly charred.
6. In a separate bowl, mix the diced cucumber, Greek yogurt, chopped dill, lemon juice, minced garlic, salt, and pepper to make the tzatziki sauce.
7. Serve the chicken skewers with the tzatziki sauce.

Ingredients:

- 4 large bell peppers, tops cut off and seeds removed
- 1/2 cup quinoa, rinsed
- 1 cup water
- 1 lb ground turkey
- 1 tbsp olive oil
- 1 small onion, diced
- 2 cloves garlic, minced
- 1 cup diced tomatoes
- 1 tsp ground cumin
- 1 tsp paprika
- 1/2 tsp salt
- 1/4 tsp black pepper
- 1/2 cup shredded low-fat cheddar cheese
- Cooking spray

Nutritional Information (per serving)

- » Calories: 300
- » Carbohydrates: 20g
- » Protein: 26g
- » Fat: 14g
- » Fiber: 4g
- » Sugars: 7g

Instructions:

1. Preheat your air fryer to 350°F.
2. In a small saucepan, bring the quinoa and water to a boil. Reduce heat, cover, and simmer for 15 minutes, or until the quinoa is cooked and water is absorbed.
3. In a skillet, heat the olive oil over medium heat. Add the diced onion and minced garlic, cooking until soft.
4. Add the ground turkey, breaking it up with a spoon, and cook until browned. Stir in the diced tomatoes, cooked quinoa, ground cumin, paprika, salt, and black pepper. Cook for another 5 minutes.
5. Stuff the bell peppers with the turkey-quinoa mixture and sprinkle shredded cheddar cheese on top.
6. Spray the air fryer basket with cooking spray and place the stuffed bell peppers in a single layer.
7. Air fry for 15-20 minutes or until the peppers are tender and the cheese is melted and bubbly.
8. Serve immediately.

4. Southwest Black Bean and Corn Salad

Ingredients:
- 1 can black beans (15 oz), drained and rinsed
- 1 cup corn kernels (fresh or frozen)
- 1 red bell pepper, diced
- 1/2 red onion, diced
- 1 avocado, diced
- 1/4 cup fresh cilantro, chopped
- 2 tbsp olive oil
- 2 tbsp lime juice
- 1 tsp ground cumin
- 1/2 tsp chili powder
- Salt and pepper to taste

Nutritional Information (per serving)
- » Calories: 220
- » Carbohydrates: 28g
- » Protein: 6g
- » Fat: 12g
- » Fiber: 9g
- » Sugars: 4g

Instructions:
1. In a large bowl, combine the black beans, corn kernels, diced red bell pepper, diced red onion, diced avocado, and chopped cilantro.
2. In a small bowl, whisk together the olive oil, lime juice, ground cumin, chili powder, salt, and pepper.
3. Pour the dressing over the salad and toss to coat.
4. Serve immediately or refrigerate for later.

5. BBQ Turkey Burger Sliders with Sweet Potato Fries

Ingredients:
- 1 lb ground turkey
- 1/4 cup BBQ sauce (sugar-free)
- 1/2 cup breadcrumbs (whole wheat)
- 1/4 cup diced onions
- 1 clove garlic, minced
- 1 tsp smoked paprika
- 1/2 tsp salt
- 1/4 tsp black pepper
- 8 whole wheat slider buns
- 2 large sweet potatoes, cut into fries
- 1 tbsp olive oil
- 1/2 tsp garlic powder
- 1/2 tsp paprika
- Salt and pepper to taste
- Cooking spray

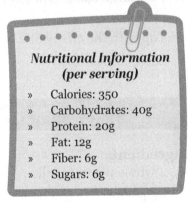

Nutritional Information (per serving)
- » Calories: 350
- » Carbohydrates: 40g
- » Protein: 20g
- » Fat: 12g
- » Fiber: 6g
- » Sugars: 6g

Instructions:
1. Preheat your air fryer to 375°F.
2. In a large bowl, combine the ground turkey, BBQ sauce, breadcrumbs, diced onions, minced garlic, smoked paprika, salt, and black pepper. Mix until well combined.
3. Form the mixture into small patties and place them in the air fryer basket, sprayed with cooking spray.
4. Air fry the turkey sliders for 10-12 minutes, flipping halfway through, until cooked through and slightly charred.
5. Meanwhile, toss the sweet potato fries with olive oil, garlic powder, paprika, salt, and pepper.
6. Place the sweet potato fries in the air fryer basket and air fry for 15-20 minutes, shaking the basket halfway through, until crispy and golden brown.
7. Serve the turkey sliders on whole wheat buns with sweet potato fries on the side.

6. Asian Sesame Ginger Tofu Salad

Ingredients:

- 1 block firm tofu, drained and cubed
- 1 tbsp soy sauce (low sodium)
- 1 tbsp sesame oil
- 1 tbsp rice vinegar
- 1 tsp grated ginger
- 1 clove garlic, minced
- 1/4 tsp red pepper flakes (optional)
- 4 cups mixed greens
- 1 cup shredded carrots
- 1 cup sliced cucumbers
- 1/4 cup sliced green onions
- 2 tbsp sesame seeds
- Cooking spray

Nutritional Information (per serving)

- » Calories: 220
- » Carbohydrates: 14g
- » Protein: 12g
- » Fat: 14g
- » Fiber: 4g
- » Sugars: 3g

Instructions:

1. Preheat your air fryer to 375°F.
2. In a bowl, whisk together the soy sauce, sesame oil, rice vinegar, grated ginger, minced garlic, and red pepper flakes.
3. Add the cubed tofu to the marinade and toss to coat. Let it marinate for at least 15 minutes.
4. Spray the air fryer basket with cooking spray and place the marinated tofu in a single layer.
5. Air fry for 10-12 minutes, shaking the basket halfway through, until the tofu is crispy and golden.
6. In a large salad bowl, combine the mixed greens, shredded carrots, sliced cucumbers, and green onions.
7. Top with the crispy tofu and sprinkle with sesame seeds.
8. Serve immediately.

7. Mediterranean Veggie Wrap with Hummus

Ingredients:

- 4 whole wheat tortillas
- 1 cup store-bought hummus
- 1 cucumber, sliced
- 1 cup cherry tomatoes, halved
- 1/2 red onion, thinly sliced
- 1/2 cup crumbled feta cheese
- 1/4 cup sliced black olives
- 2 cups mixed greens
- 1 tbsp olive oil
- 1 tbsp lemon juice
- Salt and pepper to taste

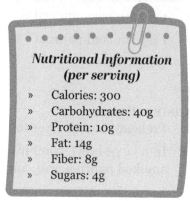

Nutritional Information (per serving)

- » Calories: 300
- » Carbohydrates: 40g
- » Protein: 10g
- » Fat: 14g
- » Fiber: 8g
- » Sugars: 4g

Instructions:

1. In a small bowl, whisk together the olive oil, lemon juice, salt, and pepper.
2. In a large bowl, toss the mixed greens with the dressing.
3. Warm the whole wheat tortillas in the air fryer for 1-2 minutes.
4. Spread hummus evenly over each tortilla.
5. Layer the dressed mixed greens, sliced cucumber, cherry tomatoes, red onion, crumbled feta cheese, and black olives on each tortilla.
6. Roll up the tortillas and serve immediately.

8. Lemon Herb Grilled Shrimp Salad

Ingredients:
- 1 lb shrimp, peeled and deveined
- 2 tbsp olive oil
- 2 tbsp lemon juice
- 2 cloves garlic, minced
- 1 tbsp chopped fresh parsley
- 1 tbsp chopped fresh dill
- Salt and pepper to taste
- 4 cups mixed greens
- 1 avocado, sliced
- 1/2 cup cherry tomatoes, halved
- 1/4 cup red onion, thinly sliced
- Cooking spray

Nutritional Information (per serving)
- » Calories: 250
- » Carbohydrates: 10g
- » Protein: 24g
- » Fat: 14g
- » Fiber: 5g
- » Sugars: 2g

Instructions:
1. Preheat your air fryer to 375°F.
2. In a bowl, mix together the olive oil, lemon juice, minced garlic, chopped parsley, chopped dill, salt, and pepper.
3. Add the shrimp and toss to coat. Let it marinate for at least 15 minutes.
4. Spray the air fryer basket with cooking spray and place the shrimp in a single layer.
5. Air fry for 6-8 minutes, shaking the basket halfway through, until the shrimp are pink and cooked through.
6. In a large salad bowl, combine the mixed greens, sliced avocado, cherry tomatoes, and red onion.
7. Top with the grilled shrimp and serve immediately.

9. Turkey and Avocado Lettuce Wraps

Ingredients:
- 8 large lettuce leaves (Romaine or Butterhead)
- 1 lb ground turkey
- 1 tbsp olive oil
- 1 small onion, diced
- 2 cloves garlic, minced
- 1 tsp ground cumin
- 1 tsp paprika
- Salt and pepper to taste
- 1 avocado, sliced
- 1/2 cup salsa (store-bought or homemade)

Nutritional Information (per serving)
- » Calories: 200
- » Carbohydrates: 8g
- » Protein: 22g
- » Fat: 10g
- » Fiber: 4g
- » Sugars: 3g

Instructions:
1. Preheat your air fryer to 375°F.
2. In a skillet, heat the olive oil over medium heat. Add the diced onion and minced garlic, cooking until soft.
3. Add the ground turkey, breaking it up with a spoon, and cook until browned. Stir in the ground cumin, paprika, salt, and pepper. Cook for another 5 minutes.
4. Place the turkey mixture in the air fryer basket and air fry for 5-7 minutes to crisp up the turkey slightly.
5. Assemble the lettuce wraps by placing the turkey mixture in each lettuce leaf and topping with sliced avocado and salsa.
6. Serve immediately.

10. Caprese Panini with Balsamic Glaze

Ingredients:
- 4 whole wheat sandwich rolls
- 2 large tomatoes, sliced
- 8 oz fresh mozzarella, sliced
- 1/4 cup fresh basil leaves
- 1 tbsp olive oil
- 2 tbsp balsamic glaze
- Salt and pepper to taste
- Cooking spray

Nutritional Information (per serving)
- » Calories: 320
- » Carbohydrates: 34g
- » Protein: 14g
- » Fat: 14g
- » Fiber: 4g
- » Sugars: 4g

Instructions:
1. Preheat your air fryer to 375°F.
2. Slice the sandwich rolls in half and lightly brush the insides with olive oil.
3. Layer the tomato slices, fresh mozzarella, and basil leaves on the bottom half of each roll. Season with salt and pepper.
4. Place the top half of the rolls on each sandwich.
5. Spray the air fryer basket with cooking spray and place the sandwiches in a single layer.
6. Air fry for 5-7 minutes, flipping halfway through, until the bread is crispy and the cheese is melted.
7. Drizzle with balsamic glaze before serving.

11. Air-Fried Falafel Pita Pockets with Tahini Sauce

Ingredients:
- 1 can chickpeas (15 oz), drained and rinsed
- 1 small onion, diced
- 2 cloves garlic, minced
- 1/4 cup fresh parsley, chopped
- 2 tbsp fresh cilantro, chopped
- 1 tsp ground cumin
- 1 tsp ground coriander
- 1/2 tsp baking powder
- 1/4 cup whole wheat flour
- Salt and pepper to taste
- 2 tbsp olive oil
- 4 whole wheat pita pockets
- 1/2 cup tahini sauce
- 1 cup chopped tomatoes
- 1 cup chopped cucumber
- Cooking spray

Nutritional Information (per serving)
- » Calories: 350
- » Carbohydrates: 45g
- » Protein: 12g
- » Fat: 14g
- » Fiber: 10g
- » Sugars: 3g

Instructions:
1. Preheat your air fryer to 375°F.
2. In a food processor, combine the chickpeas, diced onion, minced garlic, fresh parsley, fresh cilantro, ground cumin, ground coriander, baking powder, whole wheat flour, salt, and pepper. Pulse until the mixture is well combined but not completely smooth.
3. Form the mixture into small patties and place them on a plate.
4. Spray the air fryer basket with cooking spray and place the falafel patties in a single layer.
5. Air fry for 10-12 minutes, flipping halfway through, until the falafel is golden and crispy.
6. Warm the whole wheat pita pockets in the air fryer for 1-2 minutes.
7. Fill each pita pocket with falafel, chopped tomatoes, and chopped cucumber. Drizzle with tahini sauce.
8. Serve immediately.

12. Salmon Nicoise Salad with Dijon Dressing

Ingredients:
- 2 salmon fillets (4 oz each)
- 1 tbsp olive oil
- Salt and pepper to taste
- 4 cups mixed greens
- 1/2 cup cherry tomatoes, halved
- 1/2 cup blanched green beans
- 1/4 cup sliced red onion
- 1/4 cup pitted Kalamata olives
- 2 hard-boiled eggs, quartered
- 1/4 cup Dijon mustard
- 2 tbsp lemon juice
- 1 tbsp olive oil
- 1 tsp honey
- Salt and pepper to taste
- Cooking spray

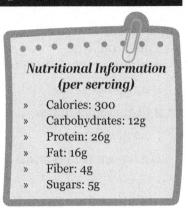

Nutritional Information (per serving)
- » Calories: 300
- » Carbohydrates: 12g
- » Protein: 26g
- » Fat: 16g
- » Fiber: 4g
- » Sugars: 5g

Instructions:
1. Preheat your air fryer to 375°F.
2. Rub the salmon fillets with olive oil and season with salt and pepper.
3. Spray the air fryer basket with cooking spray and place the salmon fillets in a single layer.
4. Air fry for 8-10 minutes, flipping halfway through, until the salmon is cooked through and flakes easily with a fork.
5. In a large salad bowl, combine the mixed greens, cherry tomatoes, blanched green beans, sliced red onion, and Kalamata olives.
6. Top with the cooked salmon fillets and quartered hard-boiled eggs.
7. In a small bowl, whisk together the Dijon mustard, lemon juice, olive oil, honey, salt, and pepper to make the dressing.
8. Drizzle the dressing over the salad and serve immediately.

13. Rainbow Veggie Buddha Bowl with Quinoa

Ingredients:
- 1 cup quinoa, rinsed
- 2 cups water
- 1 cup shredded red cabbage
- 1 cup shredded carrots
- 1 cup diced cucumber
- 1 cup cherry tomatoes, halved
- 1 avocado, sliced
- 1/4 cup fresh cilantro, chopped
- 1 tbsp olive oil
- 1 tbsp lemon juice
- 1 tbsp tahini
- 1 tsp ground cumin
- Salt and pepper to taste

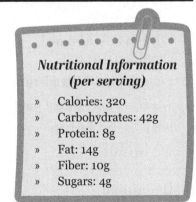

Nutritional Information (per serving)
- » Calories: 320
- » Carbohydrates: 42g
- » Protein: 8g
- » Fat: 14g
- » Fiber: 10g
- » Sugars: 4g

Instructions:
1. In a small saucepan, bring the quinoa and water to a boil. Reduce heat, cover, and simmer for 15 minutes, or until the quinoa is cooked and the water is absorbed.
2. In a large bowl, combine the shredded red cabbage, shredded carrots, diced cucumber, cherry tomatoes, sliced avocado, and chopped cilantro.
3. Add the cooked quinoa to the bowl and toss to combine.
4. In a small bowl, whisk together the olive oil, lemon juice, tahini, ground cumin, salt, and pepper to make the dressing.
5. Pour the dressing over the Buddha bowl and toss to coat.
6. Serve immediately.

14. Buffalo Cauliflower Bites with Ranch Dip

Ingredients:
- 1 medium head cauliflower, cut into florets
- 1/4 cup hot sauce
- 2 tbsp melted butter
- 1 tsp garlic powder
- 1/2 tsp smoked paprika
- 1/4 tsp salt
- 1/4 cup whole wheat flour
- 1/4 cup almond milk
- Cooking spray
- 1/2 cup ranch dressing (low-fat or sugar-free)

Nutritional Information (per serving)
- » Calories: 110
- » Carbohydrates: 14g
- » Protein: 3g
- » Fat: 6g
- » Fiber: 4g
- » Sugars: 2g

Instructions:
1. Preheat your air fryer to 400°F.
2. In a bowl, mix together the hot sauce, melted butter, garlic powder, smoked paprika, and salt.
3. In another bowl, mix together the whole wheat flour and almond milk to make a batter.
4. Dip each cauliflower floret into the batter, then coat with the hot sauce mixture.
5. Spray the air fryer basket with cooking spray and place the cauliflower florets in a single layer.
6. Air fry for 12-15 minutes, shaking the basket halfway through, until the cauliflower is crispy and golden.
7. Serve immediately with ranch dressing for dipping.

15. Air-Fried Coconut Shrimp Salad with Mango Salsa

Ingredients:
- 1 lb large shrimp, peeled and deveined
- 1/2 cup unsweetened shredded coconut
- 1/2 cup panko breadcrumbs
- 1/4 cup whole wheat flour
- 2 large eggs, beaten
- 1/2 tsp salt
- 1/4 tsp black pepper
- Cooking spray
- 4 cups mixed greens
- 1 ripe mango, diced
- 1/2 red bell pepper, diced
- 1/4 red onion, finely chopped
- 1/4 cup fresh cilantro, chopped
- 1 tbsp lime juice

Nutritional Information (per serving)
- » Calories: 350
- » Carbohydrates: 30g
- » Protein: 25g
- » Fat: 14g
- » Fiber: 6g
- » Sugars: 12g

Instructions:
1. Preheat your air fryer to 375°F.
2. In a bowl, mix together the shredded coconut, panko breadcrumbs, salt, and black pepper.
3. Place the whole wheat flour in a separate bowl and the beaten eggs in another bowl.
4. Dredge each shrimp in the flour, then dip in the eggs, and finally coat with the coconut mixture.
5. Spray the air fryer basket with cooking spray and place the shrimp in a single layer.
6. Air fry for 8-10 minutes, flipping halfway through, until the shrimp are golden and crispy.
7. In a separate bowl, mix together the diced mango, red bell pepper, red onion, chopped cilantro, and lime juice to make the mango salsa.
8. Serve the coconut shrimp over mixed greens topped with mango salsa.

16. Greek Orzo Salad with Feta and Olives

Ingredients:
- 1 cup whole wheat orzo
- 1/2 cup crumbled feta cheese
- 1/2 cup sliced Kalamata olives
- 1/2 cup diced cucumber
- 1/2 cup cherry tomatoes, halved
- 1/4 cup diced red onion
- 1/4 cup chopped fresh parsley
- 2 tbsp olive oil
- 2 tbsp red wine vinegar
- 1 tsp dried oregano
- Salt and pepper to taste

Nutritional Information (per serving)
- » Calories: 250
- » Carbohydrates: 28g
- » Protein: 8g
- » Fat: 12g
- » Fiber: 4g
- » Sugars: 4g

Instructions:
1. Cook the orzo according to package instructions. Drain and let cool.
2. In a large bowl, combine the cooked orzo, crumbled feta cheese, sliced Kalamata olives, diced cucumber, cherry tomatoes, red onion, and chopped parsley.
3. In a small bowl, whisk together the olive oil, red wine vinegar, dried oregano, salt, and pepper.
4. Pour the dressing over the salad and toss to combine.
5. Serve immediately or refrigerate for later.

17. Turkey and Cranberry Spinach Wrap

Ingredients:
- 4 whole wheat tortillas
- 1 lb cooked turkey breast, sliced
- 1/2 cup cranberry sauce (low-sugar)
- 2 cups fresh spinach leaves
- 1/4 cup crumbled goat cheese
- 1 tbsp Dijon mustard
- Salt and pepper to taste

Nutritional Information (per serving)
- » Calories: 300
- » Carbohydrates: 40g
- » Protein: 25g
- » Fat: 10g
- » Fiber: 6g
- » Sugars: 8g

Instructions:
1. Warm the whole wheat tortillas in the air fryer for 1-2 minutes.
2. Spread a thin layer of Dijon mustard on each tortilla.
3. Layer the sliced turkey breast, fresh spinach leaves, cranberry sauce, and crumbled goat cheese on each tortilla.
4. Season with salt and pepper to taste.
5. Roll up the tortillas tightly and slice in half.
6. Serve immediately.

18. Lentil and Veggie Soup with Herbed Croutons

Ingredients:
- 1 cup green lentils, rinsed
- 1 tbsp olive oil
- 1 small onion, diced
- 2 cloves garlic, minced
- 2 carrots, diced
- 2 celery stalks, diced
- 1 cup diced tomatoes
- 4 cups vegetable broth (low-sodium)
- 1 tsp dried thyme
- 1 tsp dried basil
- 1/2 tsp salt
- 1/4 tsp black pepper
- 4 slices whole grain bread, cubed
- 1 tbsp olive oil
- 1 tsp dried oregano
- Cooking spray

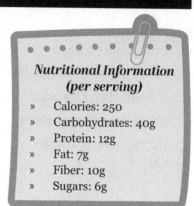

Nutritional Information (per serving)
- » Calories: 250
- » Carbohydrates: 40g
- » Protein: 12g
- » Fat: 7g
- » Fiber: 10g
- » Sugars: 6g

Instructions:
1. In a large pot, heat 1 tbsp olive oil over medium heat. Add the diced onion and minced garlic, cooking until soft.
2. Add the diced carrots and celery, cooking for another 5 minutes.
3. Stir in the green lentils, diced tomatoes, vegetable broth, dried thyme, dried basil, salt, and black pepper.
4. Bring to a boil, then reduce heat and simmer for 25-30 minutes or until the lentils are tender.
5. Meanwhile, preheat your air fryer to 375°F.
6. Toss the cubed whole grain bread with 1 tbsp olive oil and dried oregano.
7. Spray the air fryer basket with cooking spray and place the bread cubes in a single layer.
8. Air fry for 5-7 minutes, shaking the basket halfway through, until the croutons are crispy and golden.
9. Serve the soup with herbed croutons on top.

19. Shrimp and Mango Rice Paper Rolls

Ingredients:
- 1/2 lb large shrimp, cooked and peeled
- 8 rice paper wrappers
- 1 ripe mango, julienned
- 1/2 cucumber, julienned
- 1/2 cup shredded carrots
- 1/4 cup fresh mint leaves
- 1/4 cup fresh cilantro leaves
- 1/4 cup hoisin sauce (for dipping)
- 1 tbsp sesame seeds (optional)

Nutritional Information (per serving)
- » Calories: 150
- » Carbohydrates: 20g
- » Protein: 10g
- » Fat: 3g
- » Fiber: 2g
- » Sugars: 8g

Instructions:
1. Fill a large bowl with warm water. Dip one rice paper wrapper into the water for about 5 seconds to soften.
2. Lay the wrapper flat on a clean surface. In the center, place a few shrimp, julienned mango, cucumber, shredded carrots, mint leaves, and cilantro leaves.
3. Fold the sides of the wrapper over the filling, then roll tightly from the bottom up.
4. Repeat with the remaining wrappers and fillings.
5. Serve with hoisin sauce for dipping and sprinkle with sesame seeds, if desired.

Ingredients:

- 1 lb boneless, skinless chicken breasts
- 1/2 cup BBQ sauce (sugar-free)
- 2 cups cooked brown rice
- 1 cup diced pineapple
- 1/2 red bell pepper, diced
- 1/2 red onion, diced
- 1 avocado, sliced
- 2 cups mixed greens
- 1/4 cup fresh cilantro, chopped
- 1 tbsp olive oil
- Salt and pepper to taste
- Cooking spray

Nutritional Information (per serving)

- » Calories: 350
- » Carbohydrates: 40g
- » Protein: 25g
- » Fat: 12g
- » Fiber: 6g
- » Sugars: 12g

Instructions:

1. Preheat your air fryer to 375°F.
2. Rub the chicken breasts with olive oil and season with salt and pepper.
3. Spray the air fryer basket with cooking spray and place the chicken breasts in a single layer.
4. Air fry for 15-20 minutes, flipping halfway through, until the chicken is cooked through and golden brown. Brush with BBQ sauce during the last 5 minutes of cooking
5. Let the chicken rest for 5 minutes before slicing.
6. In a large salad bowl, combine the cooked brown rice, diced pineapple, red bell pepper, red onion, avocado, and mixed greens.
7. Top with the sliced BBQ chicken and sprinkle with chopped cilantro.
8. Serve immediately.

These lunch recipes are designed to be healthy, diabetic-friendly, and easy to prepare using an air fryer. Enjoy these delicious and nutritious meals to keep your blood sugar levels in check and your taste buds satisfied!

Chapter 6

Afternoon Snack Recipes

1. Ants on a Log (Celery with Peanut Butter and Raisins) .53
2. Air-Fried Ranch Zucchini Fries...................................53
3. Berry Yogurt Bark with Granola 54
4. Cinnamon Roasted Chickpea Crunch 54
5. Mini Caprese Skewers with Balsamic Glaze 55
6. Almond Butter Rice Cake Stacks with Banana 55
7. Spicy Garlic Parmesan Edamame Pods 56
8. Mango Coconut Chia Seed Pudding...........................56
9. Air-Fried Pickle Chips with Ranch Dip 57
10. Greek Yogurt Ranch Veggie Dip with Bell Pepper Slices 57
11. Tomato Basil Mozzarella Flatbread Bites 58
12. Cucumber Avocado Sushi Rolls 58
13. Greek Yogurt Blueberry Cheesecake Bites..................59
14. Crunchy Roasted Seaweed Snack Sheets 59
15. Air-Fried Artichoke Hearts with Lemon Aioli 60
16. Roasted Garlic and Herb Chickpeas 60
17. Teriyaki Tofu Rice Paper Rolls.................................61
18. Spicy Buffalo Cauliflower Bites 61
19. Almond Butter Banana Sushi Rolls...........................62
20. Air-Fried Jalapeno Poppers with Cream Cheese...........62

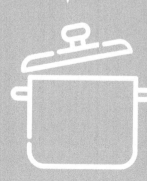

Chapter 6: Afternoon Snack Recipes

1. Ants on a Log (Celery with Peanut Butter and Raisins)

Ingredients:
- 4 celery stalks, cut into 3-inch pieces
- 1/2 cup natural peanut butter
- 1/4 cup raisins

Instructions:
1. Spread peanut butter evenly into the celery pieces.
2. Top with raisins.
3. Serve immediately.

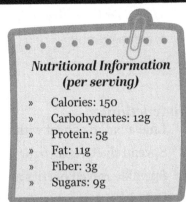

Nutritional Information (per serving)
» Calories: 150
» Carbohydrates: 12g
» Protein: 5g
» Fat: 11g
» Fiber: 3g
» Sugars: 9g

2. Air-Fried Ranch Zucchini Fries

Ingredients:
- 2 medium zucchinis, cut into sticks
- 1/2 cup whole wheat flour
- 1/2 cup almond milk
- 1/2 cup panko breadcrumbs
- 1 tbsp ranch seasoning mix
- Cooking spray

Nutritional Information (per serving)
» Calories: 120
» Carbohydrates: 20g
» Protein: 3g
» Fat: 3g
» Fiber: 4g
» Sugars: 3g

Instructions:
1. Preheat your air fryer to 400°F.
2. Dip zucchini sticks into the whole wheat flour, then almond milk, and finally coat with panko breadcrumbs mixed with ranch seasoning.
3. Spray the air fryer basket with cooking spray and place the zucchini sticks in a single layer.
4. Air fry for 10-12 minutes, shaking the basket halfway through, until golden and crispy.
5. Serve immediately.

3. Berry Yogurt Bark with Granola

Ingredients:

- 1 cup non-fat Greek yogurt
- 1/2 cup mixed berries (blueberries, raspberries, strawberries)
- 1/4 cup granola
- 1 tbsp honey

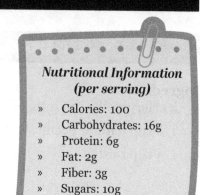

Nutritional Information (per serving)

- » Calories: 100
- » Carbohydrates: 16g
- » Protein: 6g
- » Fat: 2g
- » Fiber: 3g
- » Sugars: 10g

Instructions:

1. Line a baking sheet with parchment paper.
2. Spread the Greek yogurt evenly on the parchment paper.
3. Sprinkle mixed berries and granola on top of the yogurt.
4. Drizzle with honey.
5. Freeze for at least 2 hours or until firm.
6. Break into pieces and serve immediately.

4. Cinnamon Roasted Chickpea Crunch

Ingredients:

- 1 can chickpeas (15 oz), drained and rinsed
- 1 tbsp olive oil
- 1 tsp ground cinnamon
- 1 tbsp honey
- 1/4 tsp salt

Nutritional Information (per serving)

- » Calories: 140
- » Carbohydrates: 22g
- » Protein: 6g
- » Fat: 5g
- » Fiber: 6g
- » Sugars: 6g

Instructions:

1. Preheat your air fryer to 400°F.
2. In a bowl, toss chickpeas with olive oil, cinnamon, honey, and salt until well coated.
3. Spread chickpeas evenly in the air fryer basket.
4. Air fry for 15-20 minutes, shaking the basket halfway through, until crispy and golden.
5. Let cool completely before serving.

5. Mini Caprese Skewers with Balsamic Glaze

Ingredients:
- 1 cup cherry tomatoes
- 1/2 cup fresh mozzarella balls
- 1/4 cup fresh basil leaves
- 2 tbsp balsamic glaze
- Salt and pepper to taste

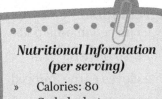

Nutritional Information
(per serving)
- » Calories: 80
- » Carbohydrates: 4g
- » Protein: 5g
- » Fat: 5g
- » Fiber: 1g
- » Sugars: 3g

Instructions:
1. Thread cherry tomatoes, mozzarella balls, and basil leaves onto small skewers.
2. Drizzle with balsamic glaze.
3. Season with salt and pepper to taste.
4. Serve immediately.

6. Almond Butter Rice Cake Stacks with Banana

Ingredients:
- 4 whole grain rice cakes
- 1/4 cup almond butter
- 2 large bananas, sliced
- 1 tbsp chia seeds
- 1 tsp ground cinnamon

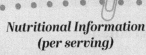

Nutritional Information
(per serving)
- » Calories: 180
- » Carbohydrates: 27g
- » Protein: 4g
- » Fat: 7g
- » Fiber: 4g
- » Sugars: 10g

Instructions:
1. Spread almond butter evenly on each rice cake.
2. Top with banana slices.
3. Sprinkle with chia seeds and ground cinnamon.
4. Serve immediately.

7. Spicy Garlic Parmesan Edamame Pods

Ingredients:
- 2 cups edamame pods
- 1 tbsp olive oil
- 2 cloves garlic, minced
- 1/4 cup grated Parmesan cheese
- 1/2 tsp red pepper flakes
- Salt to taste

Nutritional Information (per serving)
- » Calories: 150
- » Carbohydrates: 12g
- » Protein: 9g
- » Fat: 8g
- » Fiber: 4g
- » Sugars: 1g

Instructions:
1. Preheat your air fryer to 375°F.
2. In a bowl, toss edamame pods with olive oil, minced garlic, grated Parmesan cheese, red pepper flakes, and salt until well coated.
3. Spread edamame pods evenly in the air fryer basket.
4. Air fry for 8-10 minutes, shaking the basket halfway through, until crispy and golden.
5. Serve immediately.

8. Mango Coconut Chia Seed Pudding

Ingredients:
- 1 cup unsweetened coconut milk
- 1/4 cup chia seeds
- 1 ripe mango, diced
- 1 tbsp honey
- 1/2 tsp vanilla extract

Nutritional Information (per serving)
- » Calories: 180
- » Carbohydrates: 28g
- » Protein: 3g
- » Fat: 8g
- » Fiber: 8g
- » Sugars: 16g

Instructions:
1. In a bowl, mix together the coconut milk, chia seeds, honey, and vanilla extract.
2. Refrigerate for at least 4 hours or overnight until the mixture thickens.
3. Top with diced mango before serving.

9. Air-Fried Pickle Chips with Ranch Dip

Ingredients:
- 1 cup dill pickle slices
- 1/2 cup whole wheat flour
- 1/2 cup panko breadcrumbs
- 1 large egg, beaten
- 1/2 tsp garlic powder
- 1/2 tsp paprika
- Cooking spray
- 1/2 cup ranch dressing (low-fat or sugar-free)

Nutritional Information (per serving)
- » Calories: 110
- » Carbohydrates: 16g
- » Protein: 3g
- » Fat: 4g
- » Fiber: 2g
- » Sugars: 2g

Instructions:
1. Preheat your air fryer to 400°F.
2. In a bowl, mix together the whole wheat flour, garlic powder, and paprika.
3. Dip pickle slices into the flour mixture, then beaten egg, and finally coat with panko breadcrumbs.
4. Spray the air fryer basket with cooking spray and place the pickle slices in a single layer.
5. Air fry for 8-10 minutes, shaking the basket halfway through, until crispy and golden.
6. Serve with ranch dressing for dipping.

10. Greek Yogurt Ranch Veggie Dip with Bell Pepper Slices

Ingredients:
- 1 cup non-fat Greek yogurt
- 1 tbsp ranch seasoning mix
- 3 bell peppers (red, yellow, green), sliced

Instructions:
1. In a bowl, mix together the Greek yogurt and ranch seasoning mix.
2. Serve with bell pepper slices.

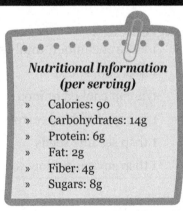

Nutritional Information (per serving)
- » Calories: 90
- » Carbohydrates: 14g
- » Protein: 6g
- » Fat: 2g
- » Fiber: 4g
- » Sugars: 8g

11. Tomato Basil Mozzarella Flatbread Bites

Ingredients:

- 2 whole wheat flatbreads
- 1 cup cherry tomatoes, halved
- 1/2 cup fresh mozzarella, sliced
- 1/4 cup fresh basil leaves
- 2 tbsp balsamic glaze
- Salt and pepper to taste
- Cooking spray

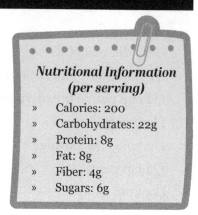

Nutritional Information (per serving)

- » Calories: 200
- » Carbohydrates: 22g
- » Protein: 8g
- » Fat: 8g
- » Fiber: 4g
- » Sugars: 6g

Instructions:

1. Preheat your air fryer to 375°F.
2. Spray the air fryer basket with cooking spray and place the whole wheat flatbreads in a single layer.
3. Top with halved cherry tomatoes, sliced mozzarella, and fresh basil leaves.
4. Air fry for 5-7 minutes or until the cheese is melted and the flatbread is crispy.
5. Drizzle with balsamic glaze and season with salt and pepper before serving.

12. Cucumber Avocado Sushi Rolls

Ingredients:

- 1 large cucumber, thinly sliced
- 1 avocado, sliced
- 1/2 cup cooked quinoa
- 1/4 cup shredded carrots
- 1 tbsp sesame seeds
- 1 tbsp soy sauce (low sodium)

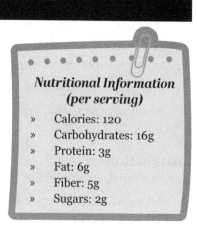

Nutritional Information (per serving)

- » Calories: 120
- » Carbohydrates: 16g
- » Protein: 3g
- » Fat: 6g
- » Fiber: 5g
- » Sugars: 2g

Instructions:

1. Lay out the cucumber slices on a flat surface.
2. Place a small amount of avocado, cooked quinoa, and shredded carrots at one end of each cucumber slice.
3. Roll up tightly and secure with a toothpick if necessary.
4. Sprinkle with sesame seeds and serve with soy sauce.

13. Greek Yogurt Blueberry Cheesecake Bites

Ingredients:
- 1 cup non-fat Greek yogurt
- 1/2 cup fresh blueberries
- 2 tbsp honey
- 1 tsp vanilla extract
- 1/4 cup graham cracker crumbs

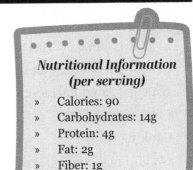

Nutritional Information (per serving)
- » Calories: 90
- » Carbohydrates: 14g
- » Protein: 4g
- » Fat: 2g
- » Fiber: 1g
- » Sugars: 10g

Instructions:
1. In a bowl, mix together the Greek yogurt, honey, and vanilla extract.
2. Spoon the mixture into a silicone mini muffin tray.
3. Top each with fresh blueberries and sprinkle with graham cracker crumbs.
4. Freeze for at least 2 hours or until firm.
5. Pop out the bites and serve immediately.

14. Crunchy Roasted Seaweed Snack Sheets

Ingredients:
- 8 sheets of nori (seaweed)
- 1 tbsp sesame oil
- 1 tsp sea salt
- Cooking spray

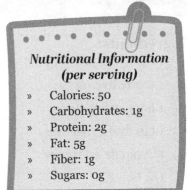

Nutritional Information (per serving)
- » Calories: 50
- » Carbohydrates: 1g
- » Protein: 2g
- » Fat: 5g
- » Fiber: 1g
- » Sugars: 0g

Instructions:
1. Preheat your air fryer to 300°F.
2. Lightly brush each nori sheet with sesame oil and sprinkle with sea salt.
3. Cut the sheets into smaller pieces if desired.
4. Spray the air fryer basket with cooking spray and place the nori sheets in a single layer.
5. Air fry for 3-5 minutes or until crispy.
6. Let cool completely before serving.

15. Air-Fried Artichoke Hearts with Lemon Aioli

Ingredients:

- 1 can artichoke hearts (14 oz), drained and halved
- 1/2 cup panko breadcrumbs
- 1/4 cup grated Parmesan cheese
- 1 large egg, beaten
- Cooking spray
- 1/4 cup mayonnaise (low-fat)
- 1 tbsp lemon juice
- 1 clove garlic, minced

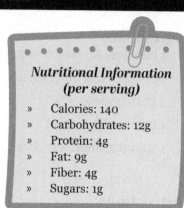

Nutritional Information (per serving)

- » Calories: 140
- » Carbohydrates: 12g
- » Protein: 4g
- » Fat: 9g
- » Fiber: 4g
- » Sugars: 1g

Instructions:

1. Preheat your air fryer to 375°F.
2. In a bowl, mix together the panko breadcrumbs and grated Parmesan cheese.
3. Dip each artichoke heart half into the beaten egg, then coat with the breadcrumb mixture.
4. Spray the air fryer basket with cooking spray and place the artichoke hearts in a single layer.
5. Air fry for 10-12 minutes, shaking the basket halfway through, until golden and crispy.
6. In a small bowl, mix together the mayonnaise, lemon juice, and minced garlic to make the lemon aioli.
7. Serve the artichoke hearts with lemon aioli for dipping.

16. Roasted Garlic and Herb Chickpeas

Ingredients:

- 1 can chickpeas (15 oz), drained and rinsed
- 1 tbsp olive oil
- 1 tsp garlic powder
- 1 tsp dried rosemary
- 1/2 tsp dried thyme
- 1/4 tsp salt
- 1/4 tsp black pepper

Nutritional Information (per serving)

- » Calories: 150
- » Carbohydrates: 22g
- » Protein: 6g
- » Fat: 5g
- » Fiber: 6g
- » Sugars: 1g

Instructions:

1. Preheat your air fryer to 400°F.
2. In a bowl, toss chickpeas with olive oil, garlic powder, dried rosemary, dried thyme, salt, and black pepper until well coated.
3. Spread chickpeas evenly in the air fryer basket.
4. Air fry for 15-20 minutes, shaking the basket halfway through, until crispy and golden.
5. Let cool completely before serving.

17. Teriyaki Tofu Rice Paper Rolls

Ingredients:
- 1 block firm tofu, drained and sliced into strips
- 8 rice paper wrappers
- 1 cup shredded carrots
- 1 cucumber, julienned
- 1/4 cup fresh mint leaves
- 1/4 cup fresh cilantro leaves
- 1/4 cup teriyaki sauce (low-sodium)
- Cooking spray

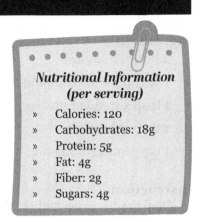

Nutritional Information (per serving)
- » Calories: 120
- » Carbohydrates: 18g
- » Protein: 5g
- » Fat: 4g
- » Fiber: 2g
- » Sugars: 4g

Instructions:
1. Preheat your air fryer to 375°F.
2. Toss tofu strips with teriyaki sauce.
3. Spray the air fryer basket with cooking spray and place the tofu strips in a single layer.
4. Air fry for 8-10 minutes, shaking the basket halfway through, until crispy and golden.
5. Fill a large bowl with warm water. Dip one rice paper wrapper into the water for about 5 seconds to soften.
6. Lay the wrapper flat on a clean surface. In the center, place a few tofu strips, shredded carrots, julienned cucumber, mint leaves, and cilantro leaves.
7. Fold the sides of the wrapper over the filling, then roll tightly from the bottom up.
8. Repeat with the remaining wrappers and fillings.
9. Serve immediately.

18. Spicy Buffalo Cauliflower Bites

Ingredients:
- 1 medium head cauliflower, cut into florets
- 1/4 cup hot sauce
- 2 tbsp melted butter
- 1 tsp garlic powder
- 1/2 tsp smoked paprika
- 1/4 tsp salt
- 1/4 cup whole wheat flour
- 1/4 cup almond milk
- Cooking spray

Nutritional Information (per serving)
- » Calories: 110
- » Carbohydrates: 14g
- » Protein: 3g
- » Fat: 6g
- » Fiber: 4g
- » Sugars: 2g

Instructions:
1. Preheat your air fryer to 400°F.
2. In a bowl, mix together the hot sauce, melted butter, garlic powder, smoked paprika, and salt.
3. In another bowl, mix together the whole wheat flour and almond milk to make a batter.
4. Dip each cauliflower floret into the batter, then coat with the hot sauce mixture.
5. Spray the air fryer basket with cooking spray and place the cauliflower florets in a single layer.
6. Air fry for 12-15 minutes, shaking the basket halfway through, until the cauliflower is crispy and golden.
7. Serve immediately.

19. Almond Butter Banana Sushi Rolls

Ingredients:
- 2 large bananas
- 1/4 cup natural almond butter
- 1 tbsp shredded unsweetened coconut
- 1 tbsp chia seeds
- 1 tsp ground cinnamon

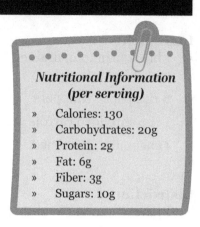

Nutritional Information (per serving)
- » Calories: 130
- » Carbohydrates: 20g
- » Protein: 2g
- » Fat: 6g
- » Fiber: 3g
- » Sugars: 10g

Instructions:
1. Peel the bananas and cut them into halves.
2. Spread almond butter evenly over each banana half.
3. Sprinkle shredded coconut, chia seeds, and ground cinnamon on top.
4. Cut the banana halves into bite-sized pieces.
5. Serve immediately.

20. Air-Fried Jalapeno Poppers with Cream Cheese

Ingredients:
- 8 large jalapenos, halved and seeds removed
- 4 oz low-fat cream cheese, softened
- 1/4 cup shredded low-fat cheddar cheese
- 1/4 tsp garlic powder
- 1/4 tsp smoked paprika
- Salt and pepper to taste
- 1/2 cup panko breadcrumbs
- 1 large egg, beaten
- Cooking spray

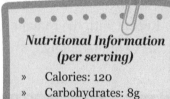

Nutritional Information (per serving)
- » Calories: 120
- » Carbohydrates: 8g
- » Protein: 4g
- » Fat: 8g
- » Fiber: 2g
- » Sugars: 2g

Instructions:
1. Preheat your air fryer to 375°F.
2. In a bowl, mix together the cream cheese, shredded cheddar cheese, garlic powder, smoked paprika, salt, and pepper until smooth.
3. Fill each jalapeno half with the cream cheese mixture.
4. Dip each filled jalapeno half into the beaten egg, then coat with panko breadcrumbs.
5. Spray the air fryer basket with cooking spray and place the jalapeno poppers in a single layer.
6. Air fry for 10-12 minutes, shaking the basket halfway through, until the jalapenos are tender and the breadcrumbs are golden.
7. Serve immediately.

These afternoon snack recipes are designed to be healthy, diabetic-friendly, and easy to prepare using an air fryer. Enjoy these delicious and nutritious snacks to keep your blood sugar levels in check and your taste buds satisfied!

Chapter 7

Dinner Recipes

1. Air-Fried Lemon Herb Chicken Thighs 64
2. Spaghetti Squash Primavera with Marinara 65
3. Honey Garlic Glazed Salmon with Broccoli 66
4. Air-Fried Stuffed Portobello Mushrooms 66
5. Turkey Meatballs with Zucchini Noodles 67
6. Coconut Curry Tofu with Jasmine Rice 68
7. Lemon Dill Shrimp Skewers with Quinoa 69
8. Greek Stuffed Bell Peppers with Ground Beef 69
9. BBQ Pulled Chicken Lettuce Wraps 70
10. Teriyaki Vegetable Stir-Fry with Brown Rice 70
11. Air-Fried Coconut Crusted Tofu with Mango Salsa 71
12. Turkey and Spinach Lasagna Roll-Ups 72
13. Mediterranean Baked Cod with Olives and Tomatoes ... 73
14. Orange Ginger Glazed Tofu with Stir-Fried Veggies 73
15. Beef and Broccoli Cauliflower Fried Rice 74
16. Cajun Blackened Shrimp Tacos with Pineapple Salsa 74
17. Air-Fried Eggplant Parmesan with Spaghetti 75
18. Pesto Zucchini Noodles with Cherry Tomatoes 75
19. Moroccan Spiced Chickpea Stew with Couscous 76
20. Air-Fried Ranch Pork Chops with Roasted Vegetables .. 77

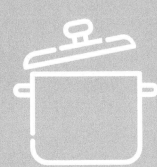

Chapter 7: Dinner Recipes

1. Air-Fried Lemon Herb Chicken Thighs

Ingredients:

- 4 bone-in, skin-on chicken thighs
- 2 tbsp olive oil
- 2 tbsp lemon juice
- 2 cloves garlic, minced
- 1 tbsp chopped fresh rosemary
- 1 tbsp chopped fresh thyme
- Salt and pepper to taste
- Cooking spray

Nutritional Information (per serving)

- » Calories: 320
- » Carbohydrates: 6g
- » Protein: 24g
- » Fat: 22g
- » Fiber: 3g
- » Sugars: 2g

Instructions:

1. Preheat your air fryer to 375°F.
2. In a bowl, mix the olive oil, lemon juice, minced garlic, chopped rosemary, chopped thyme, salt, and pepper.
3. Rub the mixture over the chicken thighs.
4. Spray the air fryer basket with cooking spray and place the chicken thighs in a single layer.
5. Air fry for 25-30 minutes, flipping halfway through, until the chicken thighs are cooked through and golden brown.
6. Serve immediately.

2. Spaghetti Squash Primavera with Marinara

Ingredients:
- 1 medium spaghetti squash
- 1 tbsp olive oil
- 1 small onion, diced
- 2 cloves garlic, minced
- 1 cup diced tomatoes
- 1 cup marinara sauce (sugar-free)
- 1/2 cup sliced bell peppers
- 1/2 cup sliced zucchini
- 1/4 cup grated Parmesan cheese
- Salt and pepper to taste
- Cooking spray

Nutritional Information (per serving)
- » Calories: 200
- » Carbohydrates: 28g
- » Protein: 6g
- » Fat: 8g
- » Fiber: 6g
- » Sugars: 12g

Instructions:
1. Preheat your air fryer to 375°F.
2. Cut the spaghetti squash in half and remove the seeds.
3. Spray the air fryer basket with cooking spray and place the spaghetti squash halves cut side down.
4. Air fry for 20-25 minutes or until the squash is tender and easily pierced with a fork.
5. Use a fork to scrape out the strands of spaghetti squash and set aside.
6. In a skillet, heat the olive oil over medium heat. Add the diced onion and minced garlic, cooking until soft.
7. Add the diced tomatoes, marinara sauce, sliced bell peppers, and sliced zucchini. Cook for 5-7 minutes or until the vegetables are tender.
8. Toss the cooked spaghetti squash with the marinara and vegetable mixture.
9. Sprinkle with grated Parmesan cheese before serving.

3. Honey Garlic Glazed Salmon with Broccoli

Ingredients:
- 2 salmon fillets (4 oz each)
- 1 tbsp honey
- 1 tbsp soy sauce (low sodium)
- 2 cloves garlic, minced
- 1/4 tsp red pepper flakes (optional)
- 2 cups broccoli florets
- 1 tbsp olive oil
- Salt and pepper to taste
- Cooking spray

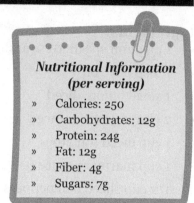

Nutritional Information (per serving)
- » Calories: 250
- » Carbohydrates: 12g
- » Protein: 24g
- » Fat: 12g
- » Fiber: 4g
- » Sugars: 7g

Instructions:
1. Preheat your air fryer to 375°F.
2. In a small bowl, mix the honey, soy sauce, minced garlic, and red pepper flakes.
3. Rub the salmon fillets with the honey garlic mixture.
4. Spray the air fryer basket with cooking spray and place the salmon fillets in a single layer.
5. In a separate bowl, toss the broccoli florets with olive oil, salt, and pepper.
6. Place the broccoli in the air fryer basket alongside the salmon.
7. Air fry for 10-12 minutes, flipping the salmon halfway through, until the salmon is cooked through and the broccoli is tender.
8. Serve immediately.

4. Air-Fried Stuffed Portobello Mushrooms

Ingredients:
- 4 large portobello mushrooms, stems removed
- 1 tbsp olive oil
- 1 small onion, diced
- 2 cloves garlic, minced
- 1 cup spinach, chopped
- 1/2 cup diced tomatoes
- 1/4 cup shredded low-fat mozzarella cheese
- Salt and pepper to taste
- Cooking spray

Nutritional Information (per serving)
- » Calories: 150
- » Carbohydrates: 10g
- » Protein: 7g
- » Fat: 10g
- » Fiber: 3g
- » Sugars: 5g

Instructions:
1. Preheat your air fryer to 375°F.
2. In a skillet, heat the olive oil over medium heat. Add the diced onion and minced garlic, cooking until soft.
3. Add the chopped spinach and diced tomatoes, cooking for another 5 minutes.
4. Season with salt and pepper.
5. Spoon the spinach mixture into the portobello mushroom caps and sprinkle with shredded mozzarella cheese.
6. Spray the air fryer basket with cooking spray and place the stuffed mushrooms in a single layer.
7. Air fry for 10-12 minutes or until the mushrooms are tender and the cheese is melted and bubbly.
8. Serve immediately.

Ingredients:
- 1 lb ground turkey
- 1/4 cup whole wheat breadcrumbs
- 1/4 cup grated Parmesan cheese
- 1 egg, beaten
- 2 cloves garlic, minced
- 1 tbsp chopped fresh parsley
- 1 tsp dried oregano
- 1/2 tsp salt
- 1/4 tsp black pepper
- 2 medium zucchinis, spiralized
- 1 tbsp olive oil
- 1 cup marinara sauce (sugar-free)
- Cooking spray

Nutritional Information (per serving)
- Calories: 280
- Carbohydrates: 15g
- Protein: 30g
- Fat: 12g
- Fiber: 4g
- Sugars: 7g

Instructions:
1. Preheat your air fryer to 375°F.
2. In a large bowl, mix together the ground turkey, whole wheat breadcrumbs, grated Parmesan cheese, beaten egg, minced garlic, chopped parsley, dried oregano, salt, and black pepper.
3. Form the mixture into meatballs and place them on a plate.
4. Spray the air fryer basket with cooking spray and place the meatballs in a single layer.
5. Air fry for 10-12 minutes, shaking the basket halfway through, until the meatballs are cooked through and golden brown.
6. In a skillet, heat the olive oil over medium heat. Add the spiralized zucchini and cook for 2-3 minutes until tender.
7. Add the marinara sauce and cooked meatballs to the skillet and toss to combine.
8. Serve immediately.

Ingredients:

- 1 block firm tofu, drained and cubed
- 1 tbsp olive oil
- 1 small onion, diced
- 2 cloves garlic, minced
- 1 tbsp grated ginger
- 1 cup coconut milk (light)
- 2 tbsp red curry paste
- 1 cup diced tomatoes
- 1 cup broccoli florets
- 1/2 cup snap peas
- 1/4 cup fresh cilantro, chopped
- 1 cup jasmine rice
- 2 cups water
- Salt and pepper to taste
- Cooking spray

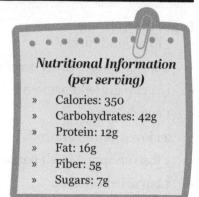

Nutritional Information (per serving)

- » Calories: 350
- » Carbohydrates: 42g
- » Protein: 12g
- » Fat: 16g
- » Fiber: 5g
- » Sugars: 7g

Instructions:

1. Preheat your air fryer to 375°F.
2. Toss the cubed tofu with olive oil, salt, and pepper.
3. Spray the air fryer basket with cooking spray and place the tofu cubes in a single layer.
4. Air fry for 10-12 minutes, shaking the basket halfway through, until the tofu is crispy and golden.
5. In a large skillet, heat 1 tbsp olive oil over medium heat. Add the diced onion, minced garlic, and grated ginger, cooking until soft.
6. Stir in the red curry paste and cook for 1-2 minutes until fragrant.
7. Add the coconut milk, diced tomatoes, broccoli florets, and snap peas. Simmer for 10-12 minutes until the vegetables are tender.
8. In a separate saucepan, bring the jasmine rice and water to a boil. Reduce heat, cover, and simmer for 15 minutes until the rice is cooked.
9. Add the crispy tofu to the curry and toss to coat.
10. Serve the coconut curry tofu over jasmine rice and sprinkle with fresh cilantro.

7. Lemon Dill Shrimp Skewers with Quinoa

Ingredients:
- 1 lb large shrimp, peeled and deveined
- 2 tbsp olive oil
- 2 tbsp lemon juice
- 2 cloves garlic, minced
- 1 tbsp chopped fresh dill
- Salt and pepper to taste
- Wooden skewers, soaked in water for 30 minutes
- 1 cup quinoa, rinsed
- 2 cups water
- 1/4 cup chopped fresh parsley
- Cooking spray

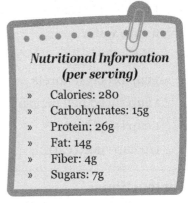

Nutritional Information (per serving)
» Calories: 300
» Carbohydrates: 28g
» Protein: 24g
» Fat: 12g
» Fiber: 4g
» Sugars: 2g

Instructions:
1. Preheat your air fryer to 375°F.
2. In a bowl, mix the olive oil, lemon juice, minced garlic,
3. chopped dill, salt, and pepper.
4. Add the shrimp and toss to coat. Let it marinate for at least 15 minutes.
5. Thread the marinated shrimp onto the soaked wooden skewers.
6. Spray the air fryer basket with cooking spray and place the shrimp skewers in a single layer.
7. Air fry for 6-8 minutes, flipping halfway through, until the shrimp are pink and cooked through.
8. In a small saucepan, bring the quinoa and water to a boil. Reduce heat, cover, and simmer for 15 minutes until the quinoa is cooked and water is absorbed.
9. Stir in the chopped parsley.
10. Serve the lemon dill shrimp skewers over quinoa.

8. Greek Stuffed Bell Peppers with Ground Beef

Ingredients:
- 4 large bell peppers, tops cut off and seeds removed
- 1 lb ground beef (lean)
- 1 tbsp olive oil
- 1 small onion, diced
- 2 cloves garlic, minced
- 1 cup diced tomatoes
- 1/2 cup cooked quinoa
- 1/4 cup crumbled feta cheese
- 1 tsp dried oregano
- 1/2 tsp ground cumin
- Salt and pepper to taste
- Cooking spray

Nutritional Information (per serving)
» Calories: 280
» Carbohydrates: 15g
» Protein: 26g
» Fat: 14g
» Fiber: 4g
» Sugars: 7g

Instructions:
1. Preheat your air fryer to 350°F.
2. In a large skillet, heat the olive oil over medium heat. Add the diced onion and minced garlic, cooking until soft.
3. Add the ground beef, breaking it up with a spoon, and cook until browned.
4. Stir in the diced tomatoes, cooked quinoa, dried oregano, ground cumin, salt, and pepper. Cook for another 5 minutes.
5. Stuff the bell peppers with the beef mixture and sprinkle crumbled feta cheese on top.
6. Spray the air fryer basket with cooking spray and place the stuffed bell peppers in a single layer.
7. Air fry for 15-20 minutes or until the peppers are tender and the cheese is melted and bubbly.
8. Serve immediately.

9. BBQ Pulled Chicken Lettuce Wraps

Ingredients:
- 1 lb boneless, skinless chicken breasts
- 1/2 cup BBQ sauce (sugar-free)
- 1/2 cup chicken broth (low sodium)
- 8 large lettuce leaves (Romaine or Butterhead)
- 1/2 red onion, thinly sliced
- 1/4 cup fresh cilantro, chopped
- Salt and pepper to taste
- Cooking spray

Nutritional Information (per serving)
- » Calories: 200
- » Carbohydrates: 10g
- » Protein: 26g
- » Fat: 6g
- » Fiber: 2g
- » Sugars: 4g

Instructions:
1. Preheat your air fryer to 375°F.
2. Place the chicken breasts in the air fryer basket, sprayed with cooking spray.
3. Air fry for 15-20 minutes, flipping halfway through, until the chicken is cooked through and tender.
4. Shred the chicken using two forks and mix with BBQ sauce and chicken broth.
5. Assemble the lettuce wraps by placing the BBQ pulled chicken in each lettuce leaf and topping with sliced red onion and chopped cilantro.
6. Serve immediately.

10. Teriyaki Vegetable Stir-Fry with Brown Rice

Ingredients:
- 1 cup brown rice
- 2 cups water
- 1 tbsp olive oil
- 1 cup broccoli florets
- 1 cup sliced bell peppers
- 1 cup snap peas
- 1/2 cup sliced carrots
- 1/4 cup teriyaki sauce (low-sodium)
- 2 tbsp soy sauce (low-sodium)
- 1 tsp grated ginger
- 1 clove garlic, minced
- 1 tbsp sesame seeds
- Cooking spray

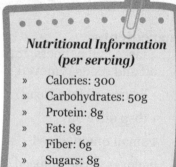

Nutritional Information (per serving)
- » Calories: 300
- » Carbohydrates: 50g
- » Protein: 8g
- » Fat: 8g
- » Fiber: 6g
- » Sugars: 8g

Instructions:
1. In a small saucepan, bring the brown rice and water to a boil. Reduce heat, cover, and simmer for 40-45 minutes, or until the rice is cooked and water is absorbed.
2. Preheat your air fryer to 375°F.
3. In a bowl, toss the broccoli florets, sliced bell peppers, snap peas, and sliced carrots with olive oil, teriyaki sauce, soy sauce, grated ginger, and minced garlic.
4. Spray the air fryer basket with cooking spray and place the vegetables in a single layer.
5. Air fry for 10-12 minutes, shaking the basket halfway through, until the vegetables are tender and slightly charred.
6. Serve the teriyaki vegetable stir-fry over cooked brown rice and sprinkle with sesame seeds.

11. Air-Fried Coconut Crusted Tofu with Mango Salsa

Ingredients:
- 1 block firm tofu, drained and cubed
- 1/2 cup unsweetened shredded coconut
- 1/2 cup panko breadcrumbs
- 1/4 cup whole wheat flour
- 2 large eggs, beaten
- 1/2 tsp salt
- 1/4 tsp black pepper
- Cooking spray
- 1 ripe mango, diced
- 1/2 red bell pepper, diced
- 1/4 red onion, finely chopped
- 1/4 cup fresh cilantro, chopped
- 1 tbsp lime juice

Nutritional Information (per serving)
- » Calories: 350
- » Carbohydrates: 30g
- » Protein: 15g
- » Fat: 18g
- » Fiber: 6g
- » Sugars: 8g

Instructions:
1. Preheat your air fryer to 375°F.
2. In a bowl, mix together the shredded coconut, panko breadcrumbs, salt, and black pepper.
3. Place the whole wheat flour in a separate bowl and the beaten eggs in another bowl.
4. Dredge each tofu cube in the flour, then dip in the eggs, and finally coat with the coconut mixture.
5. Spray the air fryer basket with cooking spray and place the tofu cubes in a single layer.
6. Air fry for 10-12 minutes, flipping halfway through, until the tofu is golden and crispy.
7. In a separate bowl, mix together the diced mango, red bell pepper, red onion, chopped cilantro, and lime juice to make the mango salsa.
8. Serve the coconut crusted tofu with mango salsa.

Ingredients:

- 8 lasagna noodles
- 1 lb ground turkey
- 1 tbsp olive oil
- 1 small onion, diced
- 2 cloves garlic, minced
- 1 cup ricotta cheese (low-fat)
- 1 cup fresh spinach, chopped
- 1 egg, beaten
- 1 cup marinara sauce (sugar-free)
- 1/2 cup shredded mozzarella cheese (low-fat)
- 1/4 cup grated Parmesan cheese
- 1 tsp dried oregano
- Salt and pepper to taste
- Cooking spray

Nutritional Information (per serving)

- » Calories: 350
- » Carbohydrates: 28g
- » Protein: 30g
- » Fat: 14g
- » Fiber: 4g
- » Sugars: 6g

Instructions:

1. Preheat your air fryer to 375°F.
2. Cook the lasagna noodles according to package instructions. Drain and set aside.
3. In a large skillet, heat the olive oil over medium heat. Add the diced onion and minced garlic, cooking until soft.
4. Add the ground turkey, breaking it up with a spoon, and cook until browned.
5. Stir in the chopped spinach and cook until wilted. Season with salt, pepper, and dried oregano.
6. In a bowl, mix together the ricotta cheese, beaten egg, and half of the Parmesan cheese.
7. Lay out each lasagna noodle and spread a layer of the ricotta mixture followed by the turkey-spinach mixture. Roll up each noodle and place them seam side down in the air fryer basket.
8. Top with marinara sauce and shredded mozzarella cheese.
9. Air fry for 10-12 minutes or until the cheese is melted and bubbly.
10. Sprinkle with the remaining Parmesan cheese before serving.

13. Mediterranean Baked Cod with Olives and Tomatoes

Ingredients:
- 2 cod fillets (4 oz each)
- 1 tbsp olive oil
- 1 cup cherry tomatoes, halved
- 1/4 cup pitted Kalamata olives
- 1/4 cup diced red onion
- 1 tbsp lemon juice
- 1 tbsp fresh parsley, chopped
- 1 tsp dried oregano
- Salt and pepper to taste
- Cooking spray

Nutritional Information (per serving)
- » Calories: 200
- » Carbohydrates: 8g
- » Protein: 25g
- » Fat: 8g
- » Fiber: 2g
- » Sugars: 4g

Instructions:
1. Preheat your air fryer to 375°F.
2. In a bowl, mix the olive oil, lemon juice, dried oregano, salt, and pepper.
3. Rub the mixture over the cod fillets.
4. Spray the air fryer basket with cooking spray and place the cod fillets in a single layer.
5. In a separate bowl, toss the cherry tomatoes, Kalamata olives, diced red onion, and chopped parsley.
6. Spread the tomato and olive mixture over the cod fillets.
7. Air fry for 10-12 minutes, or until the cod is cooked through and flakes easily with a fork.
8. Serve immediately.

14. Orange Ginger Glazed Tofu with Stir-Fried Veggies

Ingredients:
- 1 block firm tofu, drained and cubed
- 1/2 cup orange juice
- 1 tbsp soy sauce (low sodium)
- 1 tbsp honey
- 1 tbsp grated ginger
- 1 clove garlic, minced
- 1 tbsp olive oil
- 1 cup broccoli florets
- 1 cup snap peas
- 1/2 cup sliced carrots
- 1/4 cup sliced bell peppers
- 1 tbsp sesame seeds
- Salt and pepper to taste
- Cooking spray

Nutritional Information (per serving)
- » Calories: 250
- » Carbohydrates: 20g
- » Protein: 12g
- » Fat: 12g
- » Fiber: 5g
- » Sugars: 10g

Instructions:
1. Preheat your air fryer to 375°F.
2. In a bowl, mix together the orange juice, soy sauce, honey, grated ginger, and minced garlic.
3. Toss the cubed tofu with half of the orange ginger sauce.
4. Spray the air fryer basket with cooking spray and place the tofu cubes in a single layer.
5. Air fry for 10-12 minutes, shaking the basket halfway through, until the tofu is golden and crispy.
6. In a large skillet, heat the olive oil over medium heat. Add the broccoli florets, snap peas, sliced carrots, and sliced bell peppers. Stir-fry for 5-7 minutes until tender.
7. Add the crispy tofu and remaining orange ginger sauce to the skillet and toss to coat.
8. Sprinkle with sesame seeds before serving.

15. Beef and Broccoli Cauliflower Fried Rice

Ingredients:
- 1 lb flank steak, thinly sliced
- 1 tbsp olive oil
- 2 cloves garlic, minced
- 1 tsp grated ginger
- 1 cup broccoli florets
- 2 cups riced cauliflower
- 1/4 cup soy sauce (low sodium)
- 1 tbsp sesame oil
- 1/4 cup sliced green onions
- 1 tbsp sesame seeds
- Salt and pepper to taste
- Cooking spray

Nutritional Information (per serving)
- » Calories: 300
- » Carbohydrates: 12g
- » Protein: 25g
- » Fat: 18g
- » Fiber: 4g
- » Sugars: 4g

Instructions:
1. Preheat your air fryer to 375°F.
2. Toss the sliced flank steak with olive oil, salt, and pepper.
3. Spray the air fryer basket with cooking spray and place the steak in a single layer.
4. Air fry for 8-10 minutes, shaking the basket halfway through, until the steak is cooked to your desired doneness.
5. In a large skillet, heat the sesame oil over medium heat. Add the minced garlic and grated ginger, cooking until fragrant.
6. Add the broccoli florets and stir-fry for 3-4 minutes until tender.
7. Stir in the riced cauliflower and soy sauce, cooking for another 3-4 minutes until the cauliflower is tender.
8. Add the cooked steak to the skillet and toss to combine.
9. Sprinkle with sliced green onions and sesame seeds before serving.

16. Cajun Blackened Shrimp Tacos with Pineapple Salsa

Ingredients:
- 1 lb large shrimp, peeled and deveined
- 1 tbsp olive oil
- 1 tbsp Cajun seasoning
- 8 small whole wheat tortillas
- 1 cup diced pineapple
- 1/2 red onion, finely chopped
- 1/4 cup fresh cilantro, chopped
- 1 tbsp lime juice
- Salt and pepper to taste
- Cooking spray

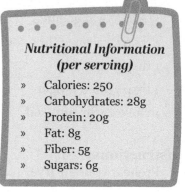

Nutritional Information (per serving)
- » Calories: 250
- » Carbohydrates: 28g
- » Protein: 20g
- » Fat: 8g
- » Fiber: 5g
- » Sugars: 6g

Instructions:
1. Preheat your air fryer to 375°F.
2. Toss the shrimp with olive oil and Cajun seasoning.
3. Spray the air fryer basket with cooking spray and place the shrimp in a single layer.
4. Air fry for 6-8 minutes, flipping halfway through, until the shrimp are pink and cooked through.
5. In a bowl, mix together the diced pineapple, red onion, chopped cilantro, lime juice, salt, and pepper to make the pineapple salsa.
6. Warm the whole wheat tortillas in the air fryer for 1-2 minutes.
7. Assemble the tacos by placing the shrimp in each tortilla and topping with pineapple salsa.
8. Serve immediately.

17. Air-Fried Eggplant Parmesan with Spaghetti

Ingredients:
- 1 large eggplant, sliced into rounds
- 1/2 cup whole wheat flour
- 2 large eggs, beaten
- 1 cup panko breadcrumbs
- 1/2 cup grated Parmesan cheese
- 1 cup marinara sauce (sugar-free)
- 1/2 cup shredded mozzarella cheese (low-fat)
- 8 oz whole wheat spaghetti
- 1 tbsp olive oil
- Salt and pepper to taste
- Cooking spray

Nutritional Information (per serving)
- » Calories: 400
- » Carbohydrates: 55g
- » Protein: 18g
- » Fat: 12g
- » Fiber: 10g
- » Sugars: 10g

Instructions:
1. Preheat your air fryer to 375°F.
2. In a bowl, mix the panko breadcrumbs and grated Parmesan cheese.
3. Dredge the eggplant slices in whole wheat flour, then dip in beaten eggs, and finally coat with the breadcrumb mixture.
4. Spray the air fryer basket with cooking spray and place the eggplant slices in a single layer.
5. Air fry for 10-12 minutes, flipping halfway through, until the eggplant is golden and crispy.
6. Meanwhile, cook the spaghetti according to package instructions. Drain and set aside.
7. In a skillet, heat the olive oil over medium heat. Add the cooked spaghetti and marinara sauce, tossing to coat.
8. Top the air-fried eggplant slices with shredded mozzarella cheese and air fry for an additional 2-3 minutes until the cheese is melted and bubbly.
9. Serve the eggplant Parmesan over the spaghetti.

18. Pesto Zucchini Noodles with Cherry Tomatoes

Ingredients:
- 2 medium zucchinis, spiralized
- 1 cup cherry tomatoes, halved
- 1/4 cup basil pesto (store-bought or homemade)
- 2 tbsp grated Parmesan cheese
- 1 tbsp olive oil
- Salt and pepper to taste
- Cooking spray

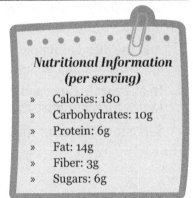

Nutritional Information (per serving)
- » Calories: 180
- » Carbohydrates: 10g
- » Protein: 6g
- » Fat: 14g
- » Fiber: 3g
- » Sugars: 6g

Instructions:
1. Preheat your air fryer to 375°F.
2. Toss the spiralized zucchini noodles with olive oil, salt, and pepper.
3. Spray the air fryer basket with cooking spray and place the zucchini noodles in a single layer.
4. Air fry for 5-7 minutes, shaking the basket halfway through, until the zucchini noodles are tender.
5. In a large bowl, toss the air-fried zucchini noodles with cherry tomatoes and basil pesto.
6. Sprinkle with grated Parmesan cheese before serving.

Ingredients:

- 1 can chickpeas (15 oz), drained and rinsed
- 1 tbsp olive oil
- 1 small onion, diced
- 2 cloves garlic, minced
- 1 cup diced tomatoes
- 1 cup vegetable broth (low-sodium)
- 1/2 cup diced carrots
- 1/2 cup diced zucchini
- 1/4 cup dried apricots, chopped
- 1 tsp ground cumin
- 1 tsp ground coriander
- 1/2 tsp ground cinnamon
- 1/4 tsp ground ginger
- Salt and pepper to taste
- 1 cup couscous
- 1 1/4 cups water
- 1/4 cup fresh cilantro, chopped

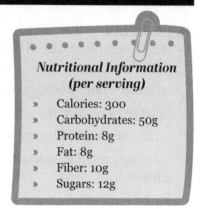

Nutritional Information (per serving)

» Calories: 300
» Carbohydrates: 50g
» Protein: 8g
» Fat: 8g
» Fiber: 10g
» Sugars: 12g

Instructions:

1. Preheat your air fryer to 375°F.
2. In a large skillet, heat the olive oil over medium heat. Add the diced onion and minced garlic, cooking until soft.
3. Stir in the ground cumin, ground coriander, ground cinnamon, and ground ginger, cooking for 1-2 minutes until fragrant.
4. Add the diced tomatoes, vegetable broth, chickpeas, diced carrots, diced zucchini, and chopped dried apricots. Simmer for 15-20 minutes until the vegetables are tender.
5. In a separate saucepan, bring the water to a boil. Stir in the couscous, cover, and remove from heat. Let sit for 5 minutes, then fluff with a fork.
6. Serve the Moroccan spiced chickpea stew over couscous and sprinkle with fresh cilantro.

Ingredients:

- 4 boneless pork chops (4 oz each)
- 1 tbsp olive oil
- 1 tbsp ranch seasoning mix
- 1/2 tsp garlic powder
- 1/2 tsp paprika
- Salt and pepper to taste
- 2 cups broccoli florets
- 2 cups diced sweet potatoes
- 1 tbsp olive oil
- 1 tsp dried thyme
- Cooking spray

Nutritional Information (per serving)

- » Calories: 350
- » Carbohydrates: 20g
- » Protein: 30g
- » Fat: 16g
- » Fiber: 6g
- » Sugars: 4g

Instructions:

1. Preheat your air fryer to 375°F.
2. In a bowl, mix the olive oil, ranch seasoning mix, garlic powder, paprika, salt, and pepper.
3. Rub the mixture over the pork chops.
4. Spray the air fryer basket with cooking spray and place the pork chops in a single layer.
5. In a separate bowl, toss the broccoli florets and diced sweet potatoes with olive oil, dried thyme, salt, and pepper.
6. Place the vegetables in the air fryer basket around the pork chops.
7. Air fry for 15-20 minutes, flipping the pork chops halfway through, until the pork chops are cooked through and the vegetables are tender.
8. Serve immediately.

These dinner recipes are designed to be healthy, diabetic-friendly, and easy to prepare using an air fryer. Enjoy these delicious and nutritious meals to keep your blood sugar levels in check and your taste buds satisfied!

Chapter 8

Dessert Recipes

1. Chocolate Avocado Mousse with Berries 79
2. Raspberry Chia Seed Pudding Parfait 79
3. Almond Flour Brownies with Walnuts 80
4. Air-Fried Cinnamon Sugar Donut Holes 80
5. Grilled Pineapple Slices with Lime Zest 81
6. Raspberry Almond Crumble Bars 81
7. Air-Fried Cinnamon Apple Slices with Yogurt Dip 82
8. Lemon Poppy Seed Muffins with Glaze 82
9. Greek Yogurt Popsicles with Mixed Berries 83
10. Chocolate Covered Strawberry Kabobs 83
11. Baked Apple Chips with Cinnamon 84
12. Coconut Flour Pumpkin Spice Cookies 84
13. Mango Coconut Rice Pudding Cups 85
14. Frozen Banana Chocolate Bites 85
15. Almond Butter Energy Balls with Dark Chocolate 86
16. Air-Fried Peach Cobbler Bites 86
17. Berry Frozen Yogurt Bark with Granola 87
18. Pistachio Cranberry Biscotti 87
19. Air-Fried Lemon Ricotta Doughnut Holes 88
20. Honey Yogurt Berry Smoothie Bowls 88

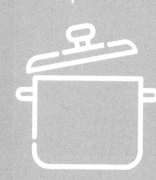

Chapter 8: Dessert Recipes

1. Chocolate Avocado Mousse with Berries

Ingredients:
- 2 ripe avocados, peeled and pitted
- 1/4 cup unsweetened cocoa powder
- 1/4 cup almond milk
- 1/4 cup honey
- 1 tsp vanilla extract
- 1 cup mixed berries (strawberries, blueberries, raspberries)

Nutritional Information (per serving)
- » Calories: 220
- » Carbohydrates: 26g
- » Protein: 3g
- » Fat: 14g
- » Fiber: 9g
- » Sugars: 18g

Instructions:
1. In a blender, combine the avocados, cocoa powder, almond milk, honey, and vanilla extract. Blend until smooth and creamy.
2. Divide the mousse into serving bowls.
3. Top with mixed berries.
4. Serve immediately or refrigerate for up to 2 hours.

2. Raspberry Chia Seed Pudding Parfait

Ingredients:
- 1 cup unsweetened almond milk
- 1/4 cup chia seeds
- 2 tbsp honey
- 1 tsp vanilla extract
- 1 cup fresh raspberries
- 1/2 cup granola (low-sugar)

Nutritional Information (per serving)
- » Calories: 200
- » Carbohydrates: 30g
- » Protein: 5g
- » Fat: 8g
- » Fiber: 11g
- » Sugars: 15g

Instructions:
1. In a bowl, mix the almond milk, chia seeds, honey, and vanilla extract.
2. Refrigerate for at least 4 hours or overnight until thickened.
3. Layer the chia pudding with fresh raspberries and granola in serving glasses.
4. Serve immediately.

3. Almond Flour Brownies with Walnuts

Ingredients:
- 1 cup almond flour
- 1/4 cup unsweetened cocoa powder
- 1/2 cup honey
- 1/4 cup coconut oil, melted
- 2 large eggs
- 1 tsp vanilla extract
- 1/2 cup chopped walnuts
- Cooking spray

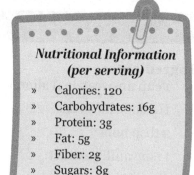

Nutritional Information (per serving)
- » Calories: 250
- » Carbohydrates: 22g
- » Protein: 6g
- » Fat: 18g
- » Fiber: 4g
- » Sugars: 16g

Instructions:
1. Preheat your air fryer to 350°F.
2. In a bowl, mix the almond flour, cocoa powder, honey, melted coconut oil, eggs, and vanilla extract until well combined.
3. Stir in the chopped walnuts.
4. Spray a small baking dish with cooking spray and pour the batter into the dish.
5. Place the dish in the air fryer and bake for 15-20 minutes or until a toothpick inserted into the center comes out clean.
6. Let cool before cutting into squares and serving.

4. Air-Fried Cinnamon Sugar Donut Holes

Ingredients:
- 1 cup whole wheat flour
- 1/4 cup almond flour
- 2 tbsp coconut sugar
- 1 tsp baking powder
- 1/2 tsp ground cinnamon
- 1/4 tsp salt
- 1/2 cup almond milk
- 1 large egg, beaten
- 2 tbsp coconut oil, melted
- 1/4 cup coconut sugar (for coating)
- 1 tsp ground cinnamon (for coating)
- Cooking spray

Nutritional Information (per serving)
- » Calories: 120
- » Carbohydrates: 16g
- » Protein: 3g
- » Fat: 5g
- » Fiber: 2g
- » Sugars: 8g

Instructions:
1. Preheat your air fryer to 350°F.
2. In a bowl, mix the whole wheat flour, almond flour, coconut sugar, baking powder, ground cinnamon, and salt.
3. Stir in the almond milk, beaten egg, and melted coconut oil until a dough forms.
4. Roll the dough into small balls and place them on a plate.
5. Spray the air fryer basket with cooking spray and place the dough balls in a single layer.
6. Air fry for 10-12 minutes or until golden brown.
7. In a small bowl, mix the coconut sugar and ground cinnamon for coating.
8. Roll the warm donut holes in the cinnamon sugar mixture.
9. Serve immediately.

5. Grilled Pineapple Slices with Lime Zest

Ingredients:
- 1 fresh pineapple, peeled, cored, and sliced into rings
- 1 tbsp honey
- 1 tsp lime zest
- Cooking spray

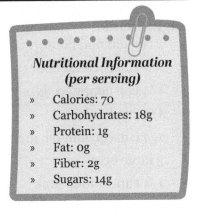

Nutritional Information (per serving)
- » Calories: 70
- » Carbohydrates: 18g
- » Protein: 1g
- » Fat: 0g
- » Fiber: 2g
- » Sugars: 14g

Instructions:
1. Preheat your air fryer to 375°F.
2. Brush the pineapple slices with honey.
3. Spray the air fryer basket with cooking spray and place the pineapple slices in a single layer.
4. Air fry for 5-7 minutes, flipping halfway through, until caramelized and golden.
5. Sprinkle with lime zest before serving.
6. Serve immediately.

6. Raspberry Almond Crumble Bars

Ingredients:
- 1 cup almond flour
- 1/2 cup rolled oats
- 1/4 cup coconut sugar
- 1/4 cup coconut oil, melted
- 1/4 cup honey
- 1 cup fresh raspberries
- 1 tsp vanilla extract
- 1/4 cup sliced almonds
- Cooking spray

Nutritional Information (per serving)
- » Calories: 200
- » Carbohydrates: 22g
- » Protein: 4g
- » Fat: 12g
- » Fiber: 4g
- » Sugars: 12g

Instructions:
1. Preheat your air fryer to 350°F.
2. In a bowl, mix the almond flour, rolled oats, coconut sugar, melted coconut oil, honey, and vanilla extract until well combined.
3. Press half of the mixture into a small baking dish sprayed with cooking spray.
4. Layer the fresh raspberries over the crust.
5. Crumble the remaining mixture on top and sprinkle with sliced almonds.
6. Place the dish in the air fryer and bake for 15-20 minutes or until golden brown.
7. Let cool before cutting into bars and serving.

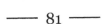

7. Lemon Poppy Seed Muffins with Glaze

Ingredients:
- 1 cup almond flour
- 1/2 cup coconut flour
- 1/4 cup poppy seeds
- 1/2 cup honey
- 1/4 cup coconut oil, melted
- 3 large eggs
- 1/4 cup almond milk
- 1 tbsp lemon zest
- 1/4 cup lemon juice
- 1 tsp baking powder
- 1/4 tsp salt
- 1/4 cup powdered erythritol (for glaze)
- 1-2 tbsp lemon juice (for glaze)
- Cooking spray

Nutritional Information (per serving)
- » Calories: 150
- » Carbohydrates: 14g
- » Protein: 4g
- » Fat: 9g
- » Fiber: 4g
- » Sugars: 8g

Instructions:
1. Preheat your air fryer to 350°F.
2. In a bowl, mix the almond flour, coconut flour, poppy seeds, baking powder, and salt.
3. In another bowl, whisk together the honey, melted coconut oil, eggs, almond milk, lemon zest, and lemon juice.
4. Combine the wet and dry ingredients and mix until well combined.
5. Spray a muffin tin with cooking spray and fill each cup with the batter.
6. Place the muffin tin in the air fryer and bake for 12-15 minutes or until a toothpick inserted into the center comes out clean.
7. Let cool before drizzling with the glaze made from powdered erythritol and lemon juice.
8. Serve immediately.

8. Air-Fried Cinnamon Apple Slices with Yogurt Dip

Ingredients:
- 2 large apples, cored and sliced
- 1 tbsp coconut sugar
- 1 tsp ground cinnamon
- 1 cup non-fat Greek yogurt
- 1 tbsp honey
- 1/2 tsp vanilla extract
- Cooking spray

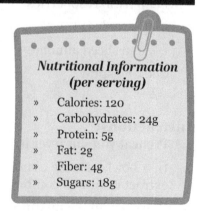

Nutritional Information (per serving)
- » Calories: 120
- » Carbohydrates: 24g
- » Protein: 5g
- » Fat: 2g
- » Fiber: 4g
- » Sugars: 18g

Instructions:
1. Preheat your air fryer to 375°F.
2. In a bowl, mix the apple slices with coconut sugar and ground cinnamon.
3. Spray the air fryer basket with cooking spray and place the apple slices in a single layer.
4. Air fry for 8-10 minutes, shaking the basket halfway through, until the apple slices are tender and slightly crispy.
5. In a small bowl, mix the Greek yogurt, honey, and vanilla extract to make the yogurt dip.
6. Serve the cinnamon apple slices with the yogurt dip.

9. Chocolate Covered Strawberry Kabobs

Ingredients:

- 1 cup fresh strawberries, hulled
- 1/2 cup dark chocolate chips (sugar-free)
- 1 tsp coconut oil
- Wooden skewers

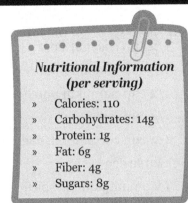

Nutritional Information (per serving)

- » Calories: 110
- » Carbohydrates: 14g
- » Protein: 1g
- » Fat: 6g
- » Fiber: 4g
- » Sugars: 8g

Instructions:

1. Thread the strawberries onto wooden skewers.
2. In a microwave-safe bowl, melt the dark chocolate chips and coconut oil in 30-second intervals, stirring in between, until smooth.
3. Dip the strawberries into the melted chocolate, coating them evenly.
4. Place the skewers on a parchment-lined baking sheet.
5. Refrigerate for 15-20 minutes or until the chocolate is set.
6. Serve immediately.

10. Greek Yogurt Popsicles with Mixed Berries

Ingredients:

- 2 cups non-fat Greek yogurt
- 1 cup mixed berries (blueberries, raspberries, strawberries)
- 2 tbsp honey
- 1 tsp vanilla extract

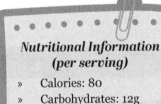

Nutritional Information (per serving)

- » Calories: 80
- » Carbohydrates: 12g
- » Protein: 6g
- » Fat: 0g
- » Fiber: 2g
- » Sugars: 10g

Instructions:

1. In a bowl, mix the Greek yogurt, honey, and vanilla extract.
2. Layer the Greek yogurt mixture and mixed berries into popsicle molds.
3. Insert popsicle sticks and freeze for at least 4 hours or until solid.
4. Serve immediately.

11. Coconut Flour Pumpkin Spice Cookies

Ingredients:
- 1/2 cup coconut flour
- 1/4 cup almond flour
- 1/2 cup pumpkin puree
- 1/4 cup honey
- 1/4 cup coconut oil, melted
- 1 large egg
- 1 tsp pumpkin pie spice
- 1/2 tsp baking powder
- 1/4 tsp salt
- Cooking spray

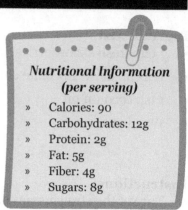

Nutritional Information (per serving)
- » Calories: 90
- » Carbohydrates: 12g
- » Protein: 2g
- » Fat: 5g
- » Fiber: 4g
- » Sugars: 8g

Instructions:
1. Preheat your air fryer to 350°F.
2. In a bowl, mix the coconut flour, almond flour, pumpkin pie spice, baking powder, and salt.
3. In another bowl, whisk together the pumpkin puree, honey, melted coconut oil, and egg.
4. Combine the wet and dry ingredients and mix until well combined.
5. Drop spoonfuls of dough onto a parchment-lined air fryer basket, sprayed with cooking spray.
6. Air fry for 8-10 minutes or until the cookies are golden and set.
7. Let cool before serving.

12. Baked Apple Chips with Cinnamon

Ingredients:
- 2 large apples, thinly sliced
- 1 tsp ground cinnamon
- Cooking spray

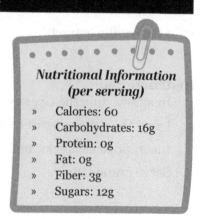

Nutritional Information (per serving)
- » Calories: 60
- » Carbohydrates: 16g
- » Protein: 0g
- » Fat: 0g
- » Fiber: 3g
- » Sugars: 12g

Instructions:
1. Preheat your air fryer to 300°F.
2. In a bowl, toss the apple slices with ground cinnamon.
3. Spray the air fryer basket with cooking spray and place the apple slices in a single layer.
4. Air fry for 15-20 minutes, flipping halfway through, until the apple slices are crispy.
5. Let cool completely before serving.

13. Frozen Banana Chocolate Bites

Ingredients:
- 2 large bananas, sliced
- 1/2 cup dark chocolate chips (sugar-free)
- 1 tsp coconut oil
- 1/4 cup chopped nuts (optional)

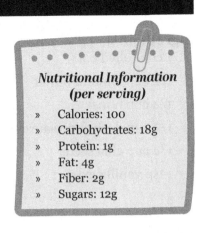

Nutritional Information (per serving)
- » Calories: 100
- » Carbohydrates: 18g
- » Protein: 1g
- » Fat: 4g
- » Fiber: 2g
- » Sugars: 12g

Instructions:
1. In a microwave-safe bowl, melt the dark chocolate chips and coconut oil in 30-second intervals, stirring in between, until smooth.
2. Dip the banana slices into the melted chocolate, coating them evenly.
3. Place the banana slices on a parchment-lined baking sheet and sprinkle with chopped nuts if desired.
4. Freeze for at least 2 hours or until solid.
5. Serve immediately.

14. Mango Coconut Rice Pudding Cups

Ingredients:
- 1/2 cup jasmine rice
- 1 cup coconut milk (light)
- 1 cup water
- 1 tbsp honey
- 1 tsp vanilla extract
- 1 ripe mango, diced

Nutritional Information (per serving)
- » Calories: 180
- » Carbohydrates: 33g
- » Protein: 3g
- » Fat: 5g
- » Fiber: 2g
- » Sugars: 15g

Instructions:
1. In a saucepan, combine the jasmine rice, coconut milk, water, honey, and vanilla extract.
2. Bring to a boil, then reduce heat and simmer for 20-25 minutes or until the rice is tender and the liquid is absorbed.
3. Divide the rice pudding into serving cups and top with diced mango.
4. Serve immediately or refrigerate for later.

15. Almond Butter Energy Balls with Dark Chocolate

Ingredients:

- 1 cup rolled oats
- 1/2 cup almond butter
- 1/4 cup honey
- 1/4 cup dark chocolate chips (sugar-free)
- 1/4 cup chia seeds
- 1 tsp vanilla extract

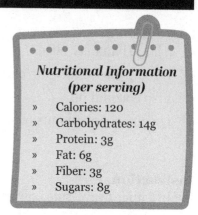

Nutritional Information (per serving)

» Calories: 120
» Carbohydrates: 14g
» Protein: 3g
» Fat: 6g
» Fiber: 3g
» Sugars: 8g

Instructions:

1. In a bowl, mix the rolled oats, almond butter, honey, dark chocolate chips, chia seeds, and vanilla extract until well combined.
2. Roll the mixture into small balls and place on a plate.
3. Refrigerate for at least 1 hour or until firm.
4. Serve immediately or store in an airtight container in the refrigerator.

16. Air-Fried Peach Cobbler Bites

Ingredients:

- 2 large peaches, peeled and diced
- 1/2 cup whole wheat flour
- 1/4 cup rolled oats
- 1/4 cup coconut sugar
- 1/4 cup coconut oil, melted
- 1 tsp ground cinnamon
- 1/2 tsp baking powder
- 1/4 tsp salt
- Cooking spray

Nutritional Information (per serving)

» Calories: 150
» Carbohydrates: 22g
» Protein: 2g
» Fat: 7g
» Fiber: 3g
» Sugars: 15g

Instructions:

1. Preheat your air fryer to 350°F.
2. In a bowl, mix the whole wheat flour, rolled oats, coconut sugar, ground cinnamon, baking powder, and salt.
3. Stir in the melted coconut oil until a crumbly mixture forms.
4. Add the diced peaches and toss to coat.
5. Spray a small baking dish with cooking spray and pour the peach mixture into the dish.
6. Place the dish in the air fryer and bake for 15-20 minutes or until golden and bubbly.
7. Let cool before serving.

17. Berry Frozen Yogurt Bark with Granola

Ingredients:
- 1 cup non-fat Greek yogurt
- 1/2 cup mixed berries (blueberries, raspberries, strawberries)
- 1/4 cup granola (low-sugar)
- 1 tbsp honey

Nutritional Information (per serving)
- » Calories: 100
- » Carbohydrates: 16g
- » Protein: 6g
- » Fat: 2g
- » Fiber: 3g
- » Sugars: 10g

Instructions:
1. Line a baking sheet with parchment paper.
2. Spread the Greek yogurt evenly on the parchment paper.
3. Sprinkle mixed berries and granola on top of the yogurt.
4. Drizzle with honey.
5. Freeze for at least 2 hours or until firm.
6. Break into pieces and serve immediately.

18. Pistachio Cranberry Biscotti

Ingredients:
- 1 cup almond flour
- 1/2 cup coconut flour
- 1/2 cup coconut sugar
- 1/2 cup chopped pistachios
- 1/2 cup dried cranberries
- 2 large eggs
- 1 tsp vanilla extract
- 1/2 tsp baking powder
- 1/4 tsp salt
- Cooking spray

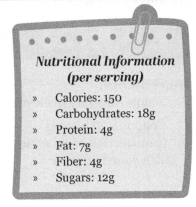

Nutritional Information (per serving)
- » Calories: 150
- » Carbohydrates: 18g
- » Protein: 4g
- » Fat: 7g
- » Fiber: 4g
- » Sugars: 12g

Instructions:
1. Preheat your air fryer to 325°F.
2. In a bowl, mix the almond flour, coconut flour, coconut sugar, chopped pistachios, dried cranberries, baking powder, and salt.
3. In another bowl, whisk together the eggs and vanilla extract.
4. Combine the wet and dry ingredients and mix until a dough forms.
5. Shape the dough into a log and place on a parchment-lined air fryer basket, sprayed with cooking spray.
6. Air fry for 20-25 minutes or until golden and firm.
7. Let cool, then slice into biscotti and air fry for an additional 5-7 minutes on each side until crispy.
8. Let cool completely before serving.

19. Air-Fried Lemon Ricotta Doughnut Holes

Ingredients:
- 1 cup whole wheat flour
- 1/4 cup almond flour
- 1/4 cup coconut sugar
- 1/2 cup ricotta cheese
- 1/4 cup almond milk
- 1 large egg, beaten
- 1 tbsp lemon zest
- 1 tsp baking powder
- 1/4 tsp salt
- 1/4 cup powdered erythritol (for coating)
- 1-2 tbsp lemon juice (for coating)
- Cooking spray

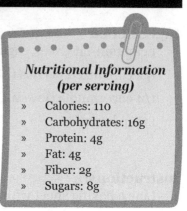

Nutritional Information (per serving)
- » Calories: 110
- » Carbohydrates: 16g
- » Protein: 4g
- » Fat: 4g
- » Fiber: 2g
- » Sugars: 8g

Instructions:
1. Preheat your air fryer to 350°F.
2. In a bowl, mix the whole wheat flour, almond flour, coconut sugar, baking powder, and salt.
3. In another bowl, whisk together the ricotta cheese, almond milk, beaten egg, and lemon zest.
4. Combine the wet and dry ingredients and mix until a dough forms.
5. Roll the dough into small balls and place them on a plate.
6. Spray the air fryer basket with cooking spray and place the dough balls in a single layer.
7. Air fry for 10-12 minutes or until golden brown.
8. In a small bowl, mix the powdered erythritol and lemon juice for coating.
9. Roll the warm doughnut holes in the lemon glaze.
10. Serve immediately.

20. Honey Yogurt Berry Smoothie Bowls

Ingredients:
- 2 cups non-fat Greek yogurt
- 1 cup mixed berries (blueberries, raspberries, strawberries)
- 1 tbsp honey
- 1/4 cup granola (low-sugar)
- 1 tbsp chia seeds
- 1 tsp vanilla extract

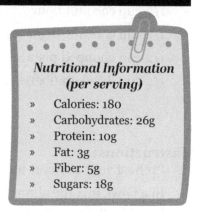

Nutritional Information (per serving)
- » Calories: 180
- » Carbohydrates: 26g
- » Protein: 10g
- » Fat: 3g
- » Fiber: 5g
- » Sugars: 18g

Instructions:
1. In a blender, mix the Greek yogurt, mixed berries, honey, and vanilla extract until smooth.
2. Pour the smoothie into bowls.
3. Top with granola and chia seeds.
4. Serve immediately.

These dessert recipes are designed to be healthy, diabetic-friendly, and easy to prepare using an air fryer. Enjoy these delicious and nutritious desserts to keep your blood sugar levels in check and your taste buds satisfied!

The Importance and Usage of a 28-Day Meal Plan for a Diabetic Air Fryer Cookbook

Managing diabetes requires careful planning, especially when it comes to diet. A 28-day meal plan tailored for diabetics using an air fryer can significantly simplify this process. It ensures a balanced intake of nutrients, helps maintain steady blood sugar levels, and makes healthy eating enjoyable and sustainable. Here's why a 28-day meal plan is essential and how to use it effectively.

Importance of a 28-Day Meal Plan

1. Blood Sugar Control: Consistency in meals helps in maintaining stable blood sugar levels. A structured meal plan eliminates guesswork and reduces the risk of blood sugar spikes.
2. Nutritional Balance: The plan ensures a balanced intake of carbohydrates, proteins, and fats. Including a variety of nutrient-dense foods helps meet the body's needs and supports overall health.
3. Portion Control: Pre-planned meals aid in managing portion sizes, crucial for weight management and diabetes control.
4. Time-Saving: A meal plan saves time on daily decision-making and grocery shopping, making it easier to stick to a healthy diet.
5. Stress Reduction: Knowing what to eat reduces stress and makes it easier to adhere to dietary recommendations.
6. Variety and Enjoyment: A diverse meal plan prevents dietary monotony and makes healthy eating more enjoyable.

How to Use the Meal Plan

1. Preparation: Review the meal plan ahead of time. Make a shopping list for the week to ensure you have all necessary ingredients.
2. Meal Prepping: Prepare ingredients in advance where possible. Chopping vegetables, marinating proteins, and preparing snacks ahead can save time during busy weekdays.
3. Flexibility: The meal plan is a guide. Feel free to swap meals or modify recipes to suit your taste and dietary needs.
4. Monitor and Adjust: Keep track of your blood sugar levels and adjust the plan if needed. Consult with a healthcare provider or dietitian to ensure the plan meets your individual health needs.
5. Stay Hydrated: Drink plenty of water throughout the day. Proper hydration supports overall health and aids in managing blood sugar levels.
6. Enjoy the Process: Cooking with an air fryer is convenient and healthy. Enjoy experimenting with different recipes and flavors.

Here's a detailed 28-day meal plan using the provided recipes in the Book:

Week 1

Day	Breakfast	Morning Snack	Lunch	Afternoon Snack	Dinner	Dessert
Day 1	Greek Yogurt Parfait with Air-Fried Granola (Page# 20)	Almond Butter Banana Bites (Page# 29)	Air-Fried Chicken Caesar Salad Wraps (Page# 40)	Air-Fried Cinnamon Pear Slices (Page# 32)	Air-Fried Lemon Herb Chicken Thighs (Page# 64)	Chocolate Avocado Mousse with Berries (Page# 79)
Day 2	Cinnamon Apple Breakfast Bites (Page# 18)	Spiced Pumpkin Seed Clusters (Page# 31)	Greek Chicken Souvlaki Skewers with Tzatziki (Page# 41)	Turkey Jerky and Cheese Stacks (Page# 33)	Spaghetti Squash Primavera with Marinara (Page# 65)	Raspberry Chia Seed Pudding Parfait (Page# 79)
Day 3	Spinach and Feta Egg Muffins (Page# 19)	Mini Bell Pepper Poppers with Cream Cheese (Page# 31)	Quinoa Stuffed Bell Peppers with Turkey (Page# 42)	Tomato Basil Mozzarella Skewers (Page# 34)	Honey Garlic Glazed Salmon with Broccoli (Page#66)	Almond Flour Brownies with Walnuts (Page#80)
Day 4	Berry Almond Breakfast Squares (Page# 19)	Air-Fried Cinnamon Pear Slices (Page# 32)	Southwest Black Bean and Corn Salad (Page#43)	Coconut Lime Energy Balls (Page#34)	Air-Fried Stuffed Portobello Mushrooms (Page#66)	Air-Fried Cinnamon Sugar Donut Holes (Page#80)
Day 5	Avocado and Egg Breakfast Boats (Page#20)	Greek Yogurt Blueberry Bark (Page# 30)	BBQ Turkey Burger Sliders with Sweet Potato Fries (Page# 43)	Honey Mustard Roasted Chickpeas (Page#35)	Turkey Meatballs with Zucchini Noodles (Page# 67)	Grilled Pineapple Slices with Lime Zest (Page# 81)
Day 6	Banana Walnut Morning Muffins (Page# 21)	Tomato Basil Mozzarella Skewers (Page# 34)	Asian Sesame Ginger Tofu Salad (Page# 44)	Apple Pie Trail Mix (Page# 35)	Coconut Curry Tofu with Jasmine Rice (Page# 68)	Raspberry Almond Crumble Bars (Page# 81)
Day 7	Zucchini and Cheese Frittata Slices (Page# 21)	Spicy Garlic Parmesan Edamame Pods (Page# 56)	Mediterranean Veggie Wrap with Hummus (Page# 44)	Air-Fried Pickle Chips with Ranch Dip (Page# 57)	Lemon Dill Shrimp Skewers with Quinoa (Page# 69)	Lemon Poppy Seed Muffins with Glaze (Page# 82)

Week 2

Day	Breakfast	Morning Snack	Lunch	Afternoon Snack	Dinner	Dessert
Day 8	Blueberry Lemon Ricotta Pancake Bites (Page# 22)	Turkey Jerky and Cheese Stacks (Page# 33)	Lemon Herb Grilled Shrimp Salad (Page# 45)	Greek Yogurt Ranch Veggie Dip with Bell Pepper Slices (Page# 57)	Greek Stuffed Bell Peppers with Ground Beef (Page# 69)	Air-Fried Cinnamon Apple Slices with Yogurt Dip (Page# 82)
Day 9	Breakfast Stuffed Bell Peppers (Page# 22)	Greek Yogurt Blueberry Cheesecake Bites (Page# 59)	Turkey and Avocado Lettuce Wraps (Page# 45)	Mango Coconut Chia Seed Pudding (Page# 56)	BBQ Pulled Chicken Lettuce Wraps (Page# 70)	Chocolate Covered Strawberry Kabobs (Page# 83)
Day 10	Air-Fried Breakfast Burrito Bowl (Page# 23)	Tomato Basil Mozzarella Skewers (Page# 34)	Caprese Panini with Balsamic Glaze (Page# 46)	Ants on a Log (Page# 53)	Teriyaki Vegetable Stir-Fry with Brown Rice (Page# 70)	Greek Yogurt Popsicles with Mixed Berries (Page# 83)
Day 11	Spinach and Mushroom Egg Cups (Page# 23)	Cinnamon Roasted Chickpea Crunch (Page# 54)	Air-Fried Falafel Pita Pockets with Tahini Sauce (Page# 46)	Cucumber Avocado Sushi Rolls (Page# 58)	Air-Fried Coconut Crusted Tofu with Mango Salsa (Page# 71)	Coconut Flour Pumpkin Spice Cookies (Page# 84)
Day 12	Peanut Butter Banana Breakfast Roll-Ups (Page# 24)	Coconut Almond Energy Bites (Page# 32)	Salmon Nicoise Salad with Dijon Dressing (Page# 47)	Crunchy Broccoli Cauliflower Bites (Page# 36)	Turkey and Spinach Lasagna Roll-Ups (Page# 72)	Baked Apple Chips with Cinnamon (Page# 84)
Day 13	Mediterranean Breakfast Pita Pockets (Page# 24)	Roasted Garlic and Herb Chickpeas (Page# 60)	Rainbow Veggie Buddha Bowl with Quinoa (Page# 47)	Air-Fried Jalapeno Poppers with Cream Cheese (Page# 62)	Mediterranean Baked Cod with Olives and Tomatoes (Page# 73)	Raspberry Almond Crumble Bars (Page# 81)
Day 14	Apple Cinnamon French Toast Sticks (Page# 25)	Crunchy Roasted Seaweed Snack Sheets (Page# 59)	Buffalo Cauliflower Bites with Ranch Dip (Page# 48)	Spicy Buffalo Cauliflower Bites (Page# 61)	Orange Ginger Glazed Tofu with Stir-Fried Veggies (Page# 73)	Mango Coconut Rice Pudding Cups (Page# 85)

Week 3

Day	Breakfast	Morning Snack	Lunch	Afternoon Snack	Dinner	Dessert
Day 15	Egg and Turkey Bacon Breakfast Tacos (Page# 25)	Almond Butter Rice Cake Stacks with Banana (Page# 55)	Air-Fried Coconut Shrimp Salad with Mango Salsa (Page# 48)	Air-Fried Ranch Zucchini Fries (Page# 53)	Beef and Broccoli Cauliflower Fried Rice (Page# 74)	Almond Butter Energy Balls with Dark Chocolate (Page# 86)
Day 16	Quinoa and Berry Breakfast Bowl (Page# 26)	Greek Yogurt Ranch Veggie Dip with Bell Pepper Slices (Page# 57)	Greek Orzo Salad with Feta and Olives (Page# 49)	Air-Fried Artichoke Hearts with Lemon Aioli (Page# 60)	Cajun Blackened Shrimp Tacos with Pineapple Salsa (Page# 74)	Air-Fried Peach Cobbler Bites (Page# 86)
Day 17	Air-Fried Breakfast Sausage Patties (Page# 26)	Honey Mustard Roasted Chickpeas (Page# 35)	Turkey and Cranberry Spinach Wrap (Page# 49)	Air-Fried Cinnamon Pear Slices (Page# 32)	Air-Fried Eggplant Parmesan with Spaghetti (Page# 75)	Berry Frozen Yogurt Bark with Granola (Page# 87)
Day 18	Veggie-Packed Breakfast Casserole Cups (Page# 27)	Tomato Basil Mozzarella Flatbread Bites (Page# 58)	Lentil and Veggie Soup with Herbed Croutons (Page# 50)	Greek Yogurt Blueberry Cheesecake Bites (Page# 59)	Pesto Zucchini Noodles with Cherry Tomatoes (Page# 75)	Pistachio Cranberry Biscotti (Page# 87)
Day 19	Protein-Packed Breakfast Sandwiches (Page# 27)	Lemon Garlic Edamame Pods (Page# 37)	Shrimp and Mango Rice Paper Rolls (Page# 50)	Almond Butter Banana Sushi Rolls (Page# 62)	Moroccan Spiced Chickpea Stew with Couscous (Page# 76)	Air-Fried Lemon Ricotta Doughnut Holes (Page# 88)
Day 20	Greek Yogurt Parfait with Air-Fried Granola (Page# 20)	Mini Caprese Skewers with Balsamic Glaze (Page# 55)	Hawaiian BBQ Chicken Salad Bowl (Page# 51)	Crunchy Cucumber Dippers with Hummus (Page# 29)	Air-Fried Ranch Pork Chops with Roasted Vegetables (Page# 77)	Honey Yogurt Berry Smoothie Bowls (Page# 88)
Day 21	Cinnamon Apple Breakfast Bites (Page# 18)	Spiced Pumpkin Seed Clusters (Page# 31)	Greek Chicken Souvlaki Skewers with Tzatziki (Page# 41)	Turkey Jerky and Cheese Stacks (Page# 33)	Spaghetti Squash Primavera with Marinara (Page# 65)	Raspberry Chia Seed Pudding Parfait (Page# 79)

Week 4

Day	Breakfast	Morning Snack	Lunch	Afternoon Snack	Dinner	Dessert
Day 22	Spinach and Feta Egg Muffins (Page# 19)	Mini Bell Pepper Poppers with Cream Cheese (Page# 31)	Quinoa Stuffed Bell Peppers with Turkey (Page# 42)	Tomato Basil Mozzarella Skewers (Page# 34)	Honey Garlic Glazed Salmon with Broccoli (Page# 66)	Almond Flour Brownies with Walnuts (Page# 80)
Day 23	Berry Almond Breakfast Squares (Page# 19)	Air-Fried Cinnamon Pear Slices (Page# 32)	Southwest Black Bean and Corn Salad (Page# 43)	Coconut Lime Energy Balls (Page# 34)	Air-Fried Stuffed Portobello Mushrooms (Page# 66)	Air-Fried Cinnamon Sugar Donut Holes (Page# 80)
Day 24	Avocado and Egg Breakfast Boats (Page# 20)	Greek Yogurt Blueberry Bark (Page# 30)	BBQ Turkey Burger Sliders with Sweet Potato Fries (Page# 43)	Honey Mustard Roasted Chickpeas (Page# 35)	Turkey Meatballs with Zucchini Noodles (Page# 67)	Grilled Pineapple Slices with Lime Zest (Page# 81)
Day 25	Banana Walnut Morning Muffins (Page# 21)	Tomato Basil Mozzarella Skewers (Page# 34)	Asian Sesame Ginger Tofu Salad (Page# 44)	Apple Pie Trail Mix (Page# 35)	Coconut Curry Tofu with Jasmine Rice (Page# 68)	Raspberry Almond Crumble Bars (Page# 81)
Day 26	Zucchini and Cheese Frittata Slices (Page# 21)	Spicy Garlic Parmesan Edamame Pods (Page# 56)	Mediterranean Veggie Wrap with Hummus (Page# 44)	Air-Fried Pickle Chips with Ranch Dip (Page# 57)	Lemon Dill Shrimp Skewers with Quinoa (Page# 69)	Lemon Poppy Seed Muffins with Glaze (Page# 82)
Day 27	Blueberry Lemon Ricotta Pancake Bites (Page# 22)	Turkey Jerky and Cheese Stacks (Page# 33)	Lemon Herb Grilled Shrimp Salad (Page# 45)	Greek Yogurt Ranch Veggie Dip with Bell Pepper Slices (Page# 57)	Greek Stuffed Bell Peppers with Ground Beef (Page# 69)	Air-Fried Cinnamon Apple Slices with Yogurt Dip (Page# 82)
Day 28	Breakfast Stuffed Bell Peppers (Page# 22)	Greek Yogurt Blueberry Cheesecake Bites (Page# 59)	Turkey and Avocado Lettuce Wraps (Page# 45)	Mango Coconut Chia Seed Pudding (Page# 56)	BBQ Pulled Chicken Lettuce Wraps (Page# 70)	Chocolate Covered Strawberry Kabobs (Page# 83)

This updated 28-day meal plan ensures all recipes included are from the provided list, making it easy for individuals with diabetes to enjoy a variety of delicious and healthy meals prepared using an air fryer.

	Week 1 Shopping List		
Produce:	5 cups spinach	2 cups cherry tomatoes	3 medium lemons
	5 bell peppers (mixed colors)	1 cup diced tomatoes	2 cups baby spinach
	2 cups mushrooms	3/4 cup diced cucumber	1/2 cup fresh parsley
	3 large apples	1/2 cup blueberries	1/4 cup chopped fresh cilantro
	2 medium zucchinis	1/2 cup raspberries	1/4 cup chopped fresh chives (optional)
	5 large bananas	1/4 cup strawberries	
	6 large avocados	1 cup mixed berries (blueberries, raspberries, strawberries)	
Dairy & Eggs:	36 large eggs	3/4 cup shredded low-fat mozzarella cheese	1 cup non-fat Greek yogurt
	1 cup skim milk	1/2 cup grated Parmesan cheese	1 cup ricotta cheese
	1 cup shredded low-fat cheddar cheese		
Bakery:	2 whole wheat tortillas	1 package whole wheat pita pockets	1 loaf whole grain bread
	4 whole grain English muffins		
Meat & Seafood:	1 lb ground turkey	1 lb ground beef	1 lb shrimp
	16 slices turkey bacon	2 lbs boneless, skinless chicken breasts	1 lb salmon fillets
Pantry:	3 cups rolled oats	1/2 cup almond milk	3 tbsp chia seeds
	2 cups almond flour	3 tsp vanilla extract	1 cup natural peanut butter
	1 cup stevia or other sugar substitute	1/2 cup chopped nuts (almonds, walnuts, or pecans)	1/2 cup hummus
	2 tsp baking powder	3 tbsp melted coconut oil	1/2 cup almond flour
	1 cup unsweetened applesauce	3 tbsp honey or sugar-free syrup	1/2 cup unsweetened applesauce

	1 cup quinoa	1/2 cup rolled oats	1/4 cup coconut flour
	1/2 cup black beans	1 cup whole wheat flour	
Canned & Packaged Goods:	1 can black beans (15 oz)	1 can diced tomatoes (15 oz)	
Spices & Seasonings:	Ground cinnamon	Dried thyme	Crushed red pepper flakes (optional)
	Garlic powder	Black pepper	Paprika
	Onion powder	Salt	Dried oregano
	Dried sage		
Frozen:	None		
Condiments:	1/2 cup guacamole		
Miscellaneous:	Cooking spray		

Week 2 Shopping List

Produce:	5 cups spinach	2 cups cherry tomatoes	3 medium lemons
	5 bell peppers (mixed colors)	1 cup diced tomatoes	2 cups baby spinach
	2 cups mushrooms	3/4 cup diced cucumber	1/2 cup fresh parsley
	3 large apples	1/2 cup blueberries	1/4 cup chopped fresh cilantro
	2 medium zucchinis	1/2 cup raspberries	1/4 cup chopped fresh chives (optional)
	5 large bananas	1/4 cup strawberries	
	6 large avocados	1 cup mixed berries (blueberries, raspberries, strawberries)	
Dairy & Eggs:	36 large eggs	3/4 cup shredded low-fat mozzarella cheese	1 cup non-fat Greek yogurt
	1 cup skim milk	1/2 cup grated Parmesan cheese	1 cup ricotta cheese
	1 cup shredded low-fat cheddar cheese		

Bakery:	2 whole wheat tortillas	1 package whole wheat pita pockets	1 loaf whole grain bread
	4 whole grain English muffins		
Meat & Seafood:	1 lb ground turkey	1 lb ground beef	1 lb shrimp
	16 slices turkey bacon	2 lbs boneless, skinless chicken breasts	1 lb salmon fillets
Pantry:	3 cups rolled oats	1/2 cup chopped nuts (almonds, walnuts, or pecans)	1/2 cup unsweetened applesauce
	2 cups almond flour	3 tbsp melted coconut oil	1 cup quinoa
	1 cup stevia or other sugar substitute	3 tbsp honey or sugar-free syrup	1/2 cup black beans
	2 tsp baking powder	3 tbsp chia seeds	1/2 cup rolled oats
	1 cup unsweetened applesauce	1 cup natural peanut butter	1 cup whole wheat flour
	1/2 cup almond milk	1/2 cup hummus	1/4 cup coconut flour
	3 tsp vanilla extract	1/2 cup almond flour	
Canned & Packaged Goods:	1 can black beans (15 oz)	1 can diced tomatoes (15 oz)	
Spices & Seasonings:	Ground cinnamon	Dried thyme	Crushed red pepper flakes (optional)
	Garlic powder	Black pepper	Paprika
	Onion powder	Salt	Dried oregano
	Dried sage		
Frozen:	None		
Condiments:	1/2 cup guacamole		
Miscellaneous:	Cooking spray		

Week 3 Shopping List

Produce:	5 cups spinach	2 cups cherry tomatoes	3 medium lemons
	5 bell peppers (mixed colors)	1 cup diced tomatoes	2 cups baby spinach
	2 cups mushrooms	3/4 cup diced cucumber	1/2 cup fresh parsley
	3 large apples	1/2 cup blueberries	1/4 cup chopped fresh cilantro
	2 medium zucchinis	1/2 cup raspberries	1/4 cup chopped fresh chives (optional)
	5 large bananas	1/4 cup strawberries	
	6 large avocados	1 cup mixed berries (blueberries, raspberries, strawberries)	
Dairy & Eggs:	36 large eggs	3/4 cup shredded low-fat mozzarella cheese	1 cup non-fat Greek yogurt
	1 cup skim milk	1/2 cup grated Parmesan cheese	1 cup ricotta cheese
	1 cup shredded low-fat cheddar cheese		
Bakery:	2 whole wheat tortillas	1 package whole wheat pita pockets	1 loaf whole grain bread
	4 whole grain English muffins		
Meat & Seafood:	1 lb ground turkey	1 lb ground beef	1 lb shrimp
	16 slices turkey bacon	2 lbs boneless, skinless chicken breasts	1 lb salmon fillets
Pantry:	3 cups rolled oats	1/2 cup almond milk	3 tbsp chia seeds
	2 cups almond flour	3 tsp vanilla extract	1 cup natural peanut butter
	1 cup stevia or other sugar substitute	1/2 cup chopped nuts (almonds, walnuts, or pecans)	1/2 cup hummus
	2 tsp baking powder	3 tbsp melted coconut oil	1/2 cup almond flour
	1 cup unsweetened applesauce	3 tbsp honey or sugar-free syrup	1/2 cup unsweetened applesauce

	1 cup quinoa	1/2 cup rolled oats	1/4 cup coconut flour
	1/2 cup black beans	1 cup whole wheat flour	
Canned & Packaged Goods:	1 can black beans (15 oz)	1 can diced tomatoes (15 oz)	
Spices & Seasonings:	Ground cinnamon	Dried thyme	Crushed red pepper flakes (optional)
	Garlic powder	Black pepper	Paprika
	Onion powder	Salt	Dried oregano
	Dried sage		
Frozen:	None		
Condiments:	1/2 cup guacamole		
Miscellaneous:	Cooking spray		

Week 4 Shopping List			
Produce:	5 cups spinach	2 cups cherry tomatoes	3 medium lemons
	5 bell peppers (mixed colors)	1 cup diced tomatoes	2 cups baby spinach
	2 cups mushrooms	3/4 cup diced cucumber	1/2 cup fresh parsley
	3 large apples	1/2 cup blueberries	1/4 cup chopped fresh cilantro
	2 medium zucchinis	1/2 cup raspberries	1/4 cup chopped fresh chives (optional)
	5 large bananas	1/4 cup strawberries	
	6 large avocados	1 cup mixed berries (blueberries, raspberries, strawberries)	
Dairy & Eggs:	36 large eggs	3/4 cup shredded low-fat mozzarella cheese	1 cup non-fat Greek yogurt
	1 cup skim milk	1/2 cup grated Parmesan cheese	1 cup ricotta cheese
	1 cup shredded low-fat cheddar cheese		

Bakery:	2 whole wheat tortillas	1 package whole wheat pita pockets	1 loaf whole grain bread
	4 whole grain English muffins		
Meat & Seafood:	1 lb ground turkey	1 lb ground beef	1 lb shrimp
	16 slices turkey bacon	2 lbs boneless, skinless chicken breasts	1 lb salmon fillets
Pantry:	3 cups rolled oats	1/2 cup chopped nuts (almonds, walnuts, or pecans)	1/2 cup unsweetened applesauce
	2 cups almond flour	3 tbsp melted coconut oil	1 cup quinoa
	1 cup stevia or other sugar sub-stitute	3 tbsp honey or sugar-free syrup	1/2 cup black beans
	2 tsp baking powder	3 tbsp chia seeds	1/2 cup rolled oats
	1 cup unsweetened applesauce	1 cup natural peanut butter	1 cup whole wheat flour
	1/2 cup almond milk	1/2 cup hummus	1/4 cup coconut flour
	3 tsp vanilla extract	1/2 cup almond flour	
Canned & Packaged Goods:	1 can black beans (15 oz)	1 can diced tomatoes (15 oz)	
Spices & Seasonings:	Ground cinnamon	Dried thyme	Crushed red pepper flakes (op-tional)
	Garlic powder	Black pepper	Paprika
	Onion powder	Salt	Dried oregano
	Dried sage		
Frozen:	None		
Condiments:	1/2 cup guacamole		
Miscellaneous:	Cooking spray		

Conclusion

Diabetic Air Fryer Cookbook 2024: 1700 Days of Easy, Healthy Low-Fat Recipes for Type 1 & 2 Diabetes with a 28-Day Meal Plan and 4-Weeks Shopping List** has been designed to empower you with the tools and knowledge needed to manage diabetes effectively while enjoying delicious and nutritious meals. This comprehensive guide is more than just a collection of recipes; it is a blueprint for a healthier lifestyle that integrates the benefits of air frying with diabetes-friendly meal planning.

Embracing a Healthier Lifestyle

One of the most significant challenges for individuals with diabetes is maintaining a diet that balances nutritional needs with flavor and variety. This cookbook addresses this challenge head-on by providing a diverse array of recipes that are both delicious and diabetes-friendly. By leveraging the air fryer, you can enjoy crispy, flavorful dishes with significantly less fat and calories than traditional frying methods. This not only helps in managing weight and blood sugar levels but also reduces the risk of heart disease and other complications associated with diabetes.

The Power of Meal Planning

The 28-day meal plan included in this cookbook serves as a structured yet flexible guide to help you navigate your dietary journey. By following the meal plan, you can ensure that you are consuming a balanced diet rich in essential nutrients, while also keeping your blood sugar levels stable. The meal plan incorporates a variety of meals from breakfast to dinner, along with snacks and desserts,

ensuring that you never get bored with your diet. It also helps in reducing the stress of daily meal planning and grocery shopping, making it easier to stick to a healthy eating regimen.

Benefits of Air Frying for Diabetics

Air frying is a game-changer for individuals managing diabetes. It allows you to enjoy your favorite fried foods without the excess oil and calories, making it easier to adhere to a low-fat, heart-healthy diet. The rapid air technology used in air fryers cooks food quickly and evenly, preserving nutrients while achieving a satisfying crunch. Additionally, air frying reduces the formation of harmful compounds that are typically produced during traditional frying, further contributing to overall health.

Diverse and Nutritious Recipes

The 1700 days of recipes in this cookbook span a wide range of cuisines and dietary preferences, ensuring that there is something for everyone. From hearty breakfasts and energizing snacks to satisfying dinners and indulgent desserts, each recipe has been crafted with careful attention to nutritional balance and flavor. Ingredients are chosen for their health benefits and ease of availability, ensuring that you can find everything you need at your local grocery store.

Empowering You to Take Control

Living with diabetes requires vigilance and dedication, but it doesn't mean you have to compromise on taste and enjoyment. This cookbook empowers you to take control of your health by providing the resources and knowledge necessary to make informed dietary choices. With the included tips on managing diabetes, understanding glycemic indexes, and the benefits of specific foods, you will be better equipped to tailor your diet to your individual needs.

A Community of Support

Beyond the recipes and meal plans, this cookbook aims to foster a sense of community among its readers. Managing diabetes can sometimes feel isolating, but remember that you are not alone. By sharing these recipes with family and friends, you can educate those around you and create a supportive environment that encourages healthy eating for everyone. Additionally, the success stories included in this book serve as a testament to the positive impact that a balanced, air-fried diet can have on managing diabetes.

Looking Forward

As you continue your journey with diabetes, let this cookbook be a constant companion in your kitchen. Revisit the recipes, experiment with new ingredients, and adapt the meal plans to suit your evolving tastes and needs. By consistently making healthy choices, you can improve your quality of life and reduce the risk of diabetes-related complications.

In conclusion, **Diabetic Air Fryer Cookbook 2024** is more than just a collection of recipes; it is a comprehensive guide to living well with diabetes. Embrace the delicious, nutritious meals and the positive lifestyle changes they bring. Here's to a healthier, happier you, one air-fried meal at a time.

Air Fryer Cooking Chart

Vegetables	Temp oF / oC	Time (Min)
Asparagus	400°F/200°C	7
Beet Chips	400°F/200°C	7
Broccoli (Florets)	400°F/200°C	10
Brussels Sprouts (1/2)	380°F/190°C	10
Corn on cob	380°F/190°C	10
Cabbage, Steaks	380°F/190°C	10-12
Carrots, Sliced	400°F/200°C	12
Cauliflower (Florets)	400°F/200°C	10-12
Eggplant, Chunks	400°F/200°C	10-12
Green Beans	400°F/200°C	7-10
Mushrooms	400°F/200°C	8-10
Onions, Chopped	400°F/200°C	10-15
Peppers, Chunks	400°F/200°C	12
Potato, Baby	400°F/200°C	15
Potato, Wedges	400°F/200°C	15
Potato Chips	400°F/200°C	8
Potato, Wedges	400°F/200°C	10
Pumpkin, Chunks	400°F/200°C	12-15
Radish Chips	380°F/190°C	8
Squash	400°F/200°C	12
Squash, Breaded	350°F/170°C	10
Sweet Potato, Fries	400°F/200°C	10
Tomato, Sliced	400°F/200°C	10
Zucchini, Sliced	400°F/200°C	10

Fish and Seafood	Temp oF / oC	Time (Min)
Calamari	400°F/200°C	5
Fish Fillet, 1 inch	400°F/200°C	10-12
Salmon Fillet	400°F/200°C	10-12
Scallops	380°F/190°C	5-7
Shrimp	380°F/190°C	6-8
Shrimp, Breaded	380°F/190°C	8

Meats	Temp oF / oC	Time (Min)
Bacon	380°F/190°C	10
Burgers	380°F/190°C	10
Chicken Whole	350°F/170°C	50-65
Chicken Breast	400°F/200°C	12
Chicken Drumsticks.	400°F/200°C	20-25
Chicken Wings	400°F/200°C	20-25
Chicken Tenders.	400°F/200°C	8
Chicken Thighs	400°F/200°C	20
Filet Mignon	400°F/200°C	8-14
Lamb Chops	400°F/200°C	8-12
Meatballs	400°F/200°C	6-8
Pork Chops	400°F/200°C	12-15
Pork Loin	380°F/190°C	12-18
Ribeye	400°F/200°C	8-12
Ribs	400°F/200°C	10-15
Sausages	400°F/200°C	12-15
Sirloin Steak	400°F/200°C	8-12

Snack/Dessert	Temp oF / oC	Time (Min)
Avocado Fries	380°F/190°C	8
Pineapple, Sliced	350°F/175°C	10-15
Mini Cheesecakes	350°F/175°C	10
Fried Oreos	380°F/190°C	6-8
Fried Pickles	380°F/190°C	8
Jalapenos, Stuffed	380°F/190°C	8-10
Chickpeas	350°F/175°C	15
Blooming Onion	380°F/190°C	10
Pizza	380°F/190°C	8-10
Toast	400°F/200°C	4
Hard Boiled Eggs	350°F/175°C	10-12
Soft Boiled Eggs	350°F/175°C	8-10

Frozen Foods	Temp oF / oC	Time (Min)
Chicken Nuggets	400°F/200°C	8-10
Cheese Sticks	400°F/200°C	7-10
Fish Filets	400°F/200°C	7-10
Frozen Fries	400°F/200°C	14-20
Pot Stickers	400°F/200°C	8-10

Kitchen Measurements Conversion Chart

Dry Weights

oz	🥄	☕ c	⚖ g	⚖ lb
1/2 OZ	1 tbsp	1/16 C	15 g	-
1 OZ	2 tbsp	1/8 C	28 g	-
2 OZ	4 tbsp	1/4 C	57 g	-
3 OZ	6 tbsp	1/3 C	85 g	-
4 OZ	8 tbsp	1/2 C	115 g	1/4 lb
8 OZ	16 tbsp	1 C	227 g	1/2 lb
12 OZ	24 tbsp	1 1/2 C	340 g	3/4 lb
16 OZ	32 tbsp	2 C	455 g	1 lb

Egg Timer

Soft: 5 min.

Medium: 7 min.

Hard: 9 min.

Oven Temperature

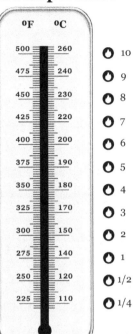

°F	°C	
500	260	🔥 10
475	240	🔥 9
450	230	🔥 8
425	220	🔥 7
400	200	🔥 6
375	190	🔥 5
350	180	🔥 4
325	170	🔥 3
300	150	🔥 2
275	140	🔥 1
250	120	🔥 1/2
225	110	🔥 1/4

Liquid Conversion

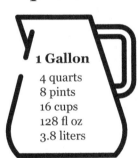

1 Gallon
4 quarts
8 pints
16 cups
128 fl oz
3.8 liters

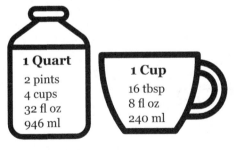

1 Quart
2 pints
4 cups
32 fl oz
946 ml

1 Cup
16 tbsp
8 fl oz
240 ml

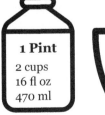

1 Pint
2 cups
16 fl oz
470 ml

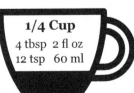

1/4 Cup
4 tbsp 2 fl oz
12 tsp 60 ml

Liquid Volumes

1 tsp = 5 ml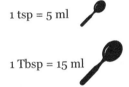

1 Tbsp = 15 ml

Dash = 1/8 tsp
Pinch = 1/16 tsp

⚖ oz	🥄	🥄	🝫 ml	☕ C	pt	qt
1 OZ	6 tsp	2 tbsp	30 ml	1/8 C	-	-
2 OZ	12 tsp	4 tbsp	60 ml	1/4 C	-	-
2 2/3 OZ	16 tsp	5 tbsp	80 ml	1/3 C	-	-
4 OZ	24 tsp	8 tbsp	120 ml	1/2 C	-	-
5 1/3 OZ	32 tsp	11 tbsp	160 ml	2/3 C	-	-
6 OZ	36 tsp	12 tbsp	177 ml	3/4 C	-	-
8 OZ	48 tsp	16 tbsp	240 ml	1 C	1/2 pt	1/4 qt
16 OZ	96 tsp	32 tbsp	470 ml	2 C	1 pt	1/2 qt
32 OZ	192 tsp	64 tbsp	950 ml	4 C	2 pt	1 qt

YOU can get this ebook for free after sending me your name and email address.

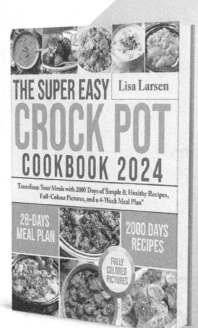

GET THIS E-BOOK FOR

FREE

YOU can get this ebook for free after sending me your name and email address.

Recipes Index

A

Air-Fried Artichoke Hearts with Lemon Aioli 60
Air-Fried Breakfast Burrito Bowl 23
Air-Fried Breakfast Sausage Patties 26
Air-Fried Chicken Caesar Salad Wraps 40
Air-Fried Cinnamon Apple Slices with Yogurt Dip 82
Air-Fried Cinnamon Pear Slices 32
Air-Fried Cinnamon Sugar Donut Holes 80
Air-Fried Coconut Crusted Tofu with Mango Salsa 71
Air-Fried Coconut Shrimp Salad with Mango Salsa 48
Air-Fried Eggplant Parmesan with Spaghetti 75
Air-Fried Falafel Pita Pockets with Tahini Sauce 46
Air-Fried Jalapeno Poppers with Cream Cheese 62
Air-Fried Lemon Herb Chicken Thighs 64
Air-Fried Lemon Ricotta Doughnut Holes 88
Air-Fried Peach Cobbler Bites 86
Air-Fried Pickle Chips with Ranch Dip 57
Air-Fried Ranch Pork Chops with Roasted Vegetables 77
Air-Fried Ranch Zucchini Fries 53
Air-Fried Stuffed Portobello Mushrooms 66
Air-Fried Veggie Omelette Cups 18
Almond Butter Banana Bites 29
Almond Butter Banana Sushi Rolls 62
Almond Butter Energy Balls with Dark Chocolate 86
Almond Butter Rice Cake Stacks with Banana 55
Almond Flour Brownies with Walnuts 80
Ants on a Log (Celery with Peanut Butter and Raisins) 53
Apple Cinnamon French Toast Sticks 25
Apple Pie Trail Mix 35
Asian Sesame Ginger Tofu Salad 44
Avocado and Egg Breakfast Boats 20

B

Baked Apple Chips with Cinnamon 84
Banana Walnut Morning Muffins 21
BBQ Pulled Chicken Lettuce Wraps 70
BBQ Turkey Burger Sliders with Sweet Potato Fries 43
Beef and Broccoli Cauliflower Fried Rice 74
Berry Almond Breakfast Squares 19
Berry Frozen Yogurt Bark with Granola 87
Berry Yogurt Bark with Granola 54
Blueberry Lemon Ricotta Pancake Bites 22
Breakfast Stuffed Bell Peppers 22
Buffalo Cauliflower Bites with Ranch Dip 48

C

Cajun Blackened Shrimp Tacos with Pineapple Salsa 74
Caprese Panini with Balsamic Glaze 46
Chocolate Avocado Mousse with Berries 79
Chocolate Covered Raspberry Clusters 33
Chocolate Covered Strawberry Kabobs 83
Cinnamon Apple Breakfast Bites 18
Cinnamon Roasted Chickpea Crunch 54
Coconut Almond Energy Bites 32
Coconut Curry Tofu with Jasmine Rice 68
Coconut Flour Pumpkin Spice Cookies 84
Coconut Lime Energy Balls 34
Cranberry Orange Almond Bars 36
Crispy Parmesan Zucchini Chips 30
Crunchy Broccoli Cauliflower Bites 36
Crunchy Cucumber Dippers with Hummus 29
Crunchy Roasted Seaweed Snack Sheets 59
Cucumber Avocado Sushi Rolls 58

E

Egg and Turkey Bacon Breakfast Tacos 25

F

Frozen Banana Chocolate Bites 85

G

Greek Chicken Souvlaki Skewers with Tzatziki 41
Greek Orzo Salad with Feta and Olives 49
Greek Stuffed Bell Peppers with Ground Beef 69
Greek Yogurt Blueberry Bark 30
Greek Yogurt Blueberry Cheesecake Bites 59
Greek Yogurt Parfait with Air-Fried Granola 20
Greek Yogurt Popsicles with Mixed Berries 83
Greek Yogurt Ranch Veggie Dip with Bell Pepper Slices 57
Grilled Pineapple Slices with Lime Zest 81

H

Hawaiian BBQ Chicken Salad Bowl 51
Honey Garlic Glazed Salmon with Broccoli 66
Honey Mustard Roasted Chickpeas 35
Honey Yogurt Berry Smoothie Bowls 88

L

Lemon Dill Shrimp Skewers with Quinoa 69
Lemon Garlic Edamame Pods 37
Lemon Herb Grilled Shrimp Salad 45
Lemon Poppy Seed Muffins with Glaze 82
Lentil and Veggie Soup with Herbed Croutons 50

M

Mango Coconut Chia Seed Pudding 56
Mango Coconut Rice Pudding Cups 85
Mediterranean Baked Cod with Olives and Tomatoes 73
Mediterranean Breakfast Pita Pockets 24
Mediterranean Veggie Wrap with Hummus 44
Mini Bell Pepper Poppers with Cream Cheese 31
Mini Caprese Skewers with Balsamic Glaze 55
Moroccan Spiced Chickpea Stew with Couscous 76

O

Orange Ginger Glazed Tofu with Stir-Fried Veggies 73

P

Peanut Butter Banana Breakfast Roll-Ups 24
Pesto Zucchini Noodles with Cherry Tomatoes 75
Pistachio Cranberry Biscotti 87
Protein-Packed Breakfast Sandwiches 27

Q

Quinoa and Berry Breakfast Bowl 26
Quinoa Stuffed Bell Peppers with Turkey 42

R

Rainbow Veggie Buddha Bowl with Quinoa 47
Raspberry Almond Crumble Bars 81

Raspberry Chia Seed Pudding Parfait 79
Roasted Beetroot Chips with Sea Salt 38
Roasted Garlic and Herb Chickpeas 60

S

Salmon Nicoise Salad with Dijon Dressing 47
Shrimp and Mango Rice Paper Rolls 50
Southwest Black Bean and Corn Salad 43
Spaghetti Squash Primavera with Marinara 65
Spiced Pumpkin Seed Clusters 31
Spicy Buffalo Cauliflower Bites 61
Spicy Garlic Parmesan Edamame Pods 56
Spinach and Feta Egg Muffins 19
Spinach and Mushroom Egg Cups 23
Sweet and Spicy Pecan Halves 38

T

Tangy Pickle Snack Sticks 37
Teriyaki Tofu Rice Paper Rolls 61
Teriyaki Vegetable Stir-Fry with Brown Rice 70
Tomato Basil Mozzarella Flatbread Bites 58
Tomato Basil Mozzarella Skewers 34
Turkey and Avocado Lettuce Wraps 45
Turkey and Cranberry Spinach Wrap 49
Turkey and Spinach Lasagna Roll-Ups 72
Turkey Jerky and Cheese Stacks 33
Turkey Meatballs with Zucchini Noodles 67

V

Veggie-Packed Breakfast Casserole Cups 27

Z

Zucchini and Cheese Frittata Slices 21

Made in the USA
Columbia, SC
05 August 2024

39975897R00059